SKIN AND CONNECTIVE TISSUE

The Human Body

Skin and Connective Tissue

Edited by Kara Rogers, Senior Editor, Biomedical Sciences

Britannica Educational Publishing
in association with
ROSEN
EDUCATIONAL SERVICES

Published in 2012 by Britannica Educational Publishing
(a trademark of Encyclopædia Britannica, Inc.)
in association with Rosen Educational Services, LLC
29 East 21st Street, New York, NY 10010.

Distributed exclusively by Rosen Educational Services.
For a listing of additional Britannica Educational Publishing titles, call toll free (800) 237-9932.

First Edition

Britannica Educational Publishing
Michael I. Levy: Executive Editor
J.E. Luebering: Senior Manager
Marilyn L. Barton: Senior Coordinator, Production Control
Steven Bosco: Director, Editorial Technologies
Lisa S. Braucher: Senior Producer and Data Editor
Yvette Charboneau: Senior Copy Editor
Kathy Nakamura: Manager, Media Acquisition
Kara Rogers: Senior Editor, Biomedical Sciences

Rosen Educational Services
Jeanne Nagle: Senior Editor
Nelson Sá: Art Director
Cindy Reiman: Photography Manager
Karen Huang: Photo Researcher
Matthew Cauli: Designer, Cover Design
Introduction by Laura Loria

Library of Congress Cataloging-in-Publication Data

Skin and connective tissue / edited by Kara Rogers.—1st ed.
p. cm.—(The human body)
"In association with Britannica Educational Publishing, Rosen Educational Services."
Includes bibliographical references and index.
ISBN 978-1-61530-656-5 (lib. bdg.)
1. Skin. 2. Connective tissues. I. Rogers, Kara.
QM481.S55 2012
612.7'92—dc23

2011013430

Manufactured in the United States of America

On the cover: Skin, represented in outline, helps protect the body's inner workings, including the calcified connective tissue of bones. *www.istockphoto.com/Aaliya Landholt*

On page x: Itself the largest organ of the human body, the skin encases and protects other vital organs. *Nacivet/Photographer's Choice/Getty Images*

On pages 1, 26, 46, 70, 90, 105, 131, 156, 178, 180, 182, 184: A three-quarter view of a bent knee revealing menisci and ligaments, two types of connective tissue. *LifeART image © 2012 Lippincott Williams & Wilkins. All rights reserved*

CONTENTS

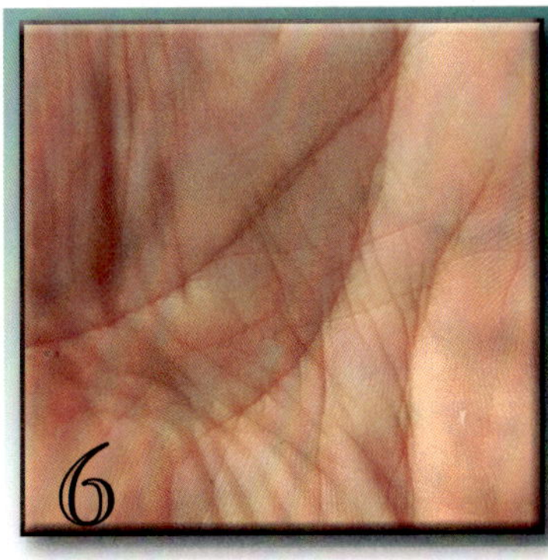

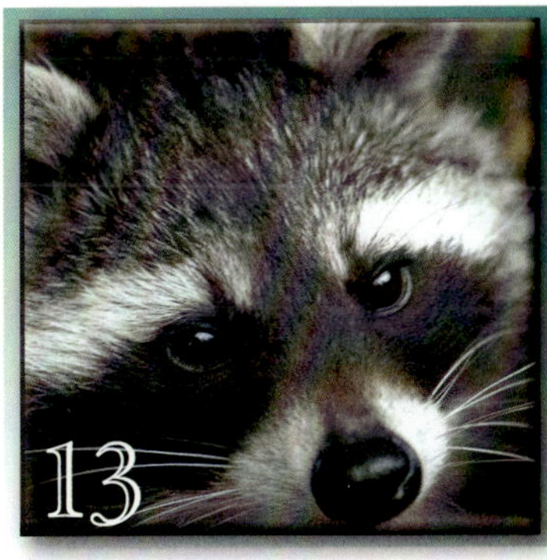

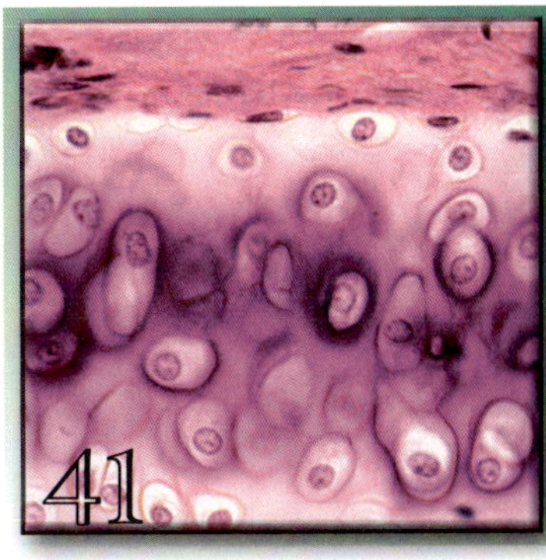

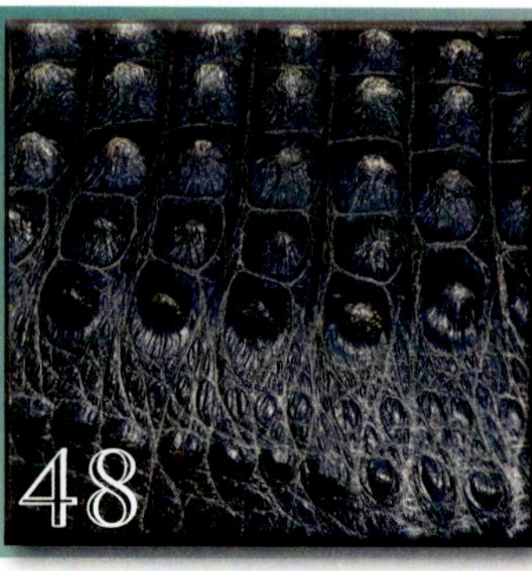
48

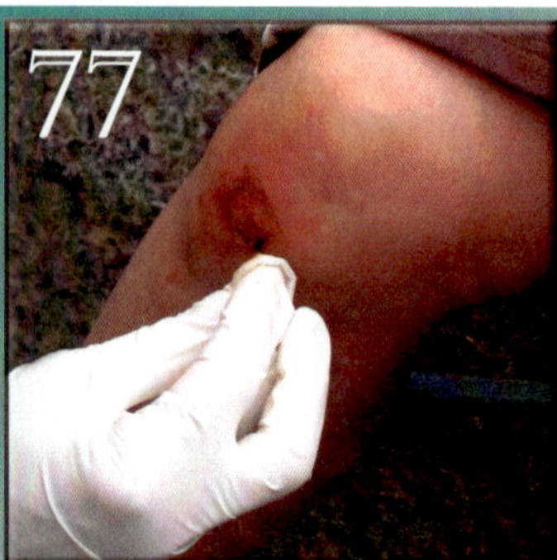
77

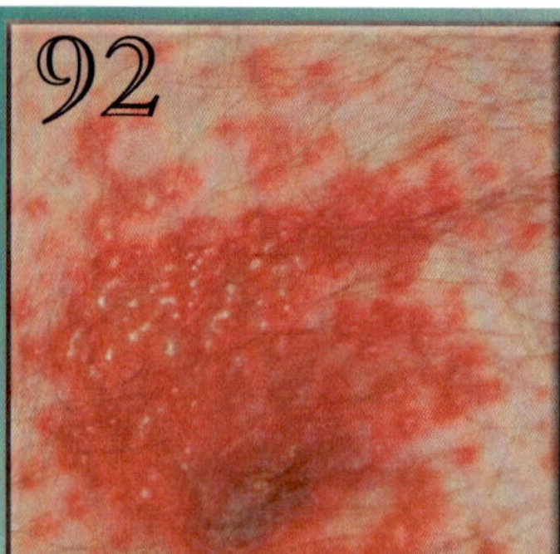
92

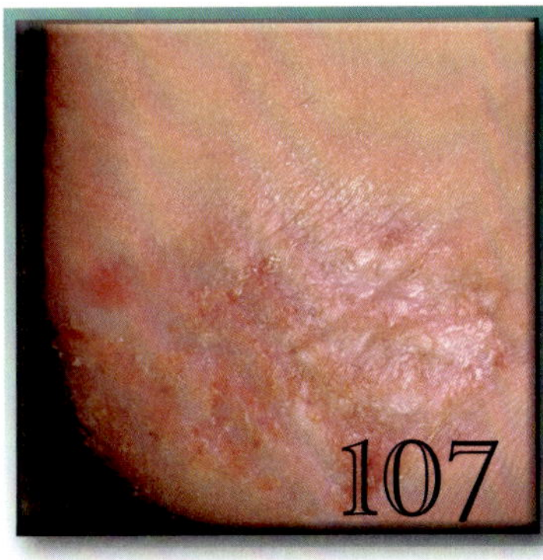
107

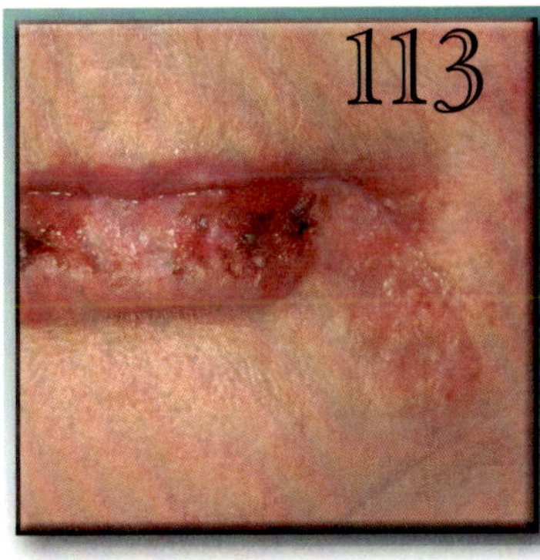
113

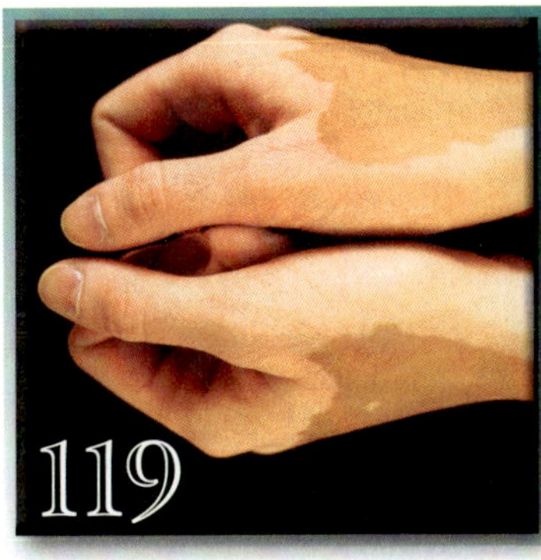
119

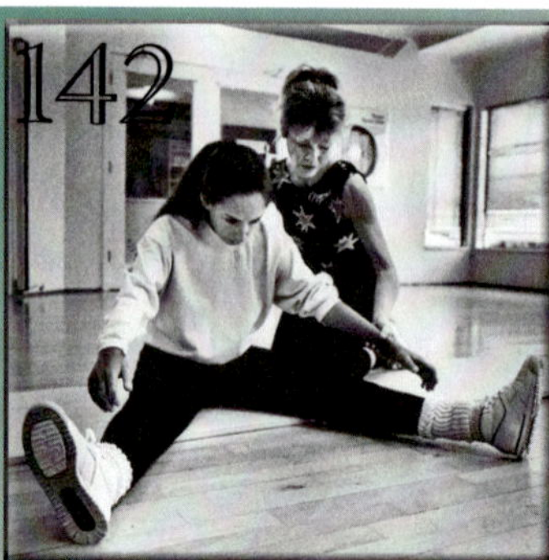
142

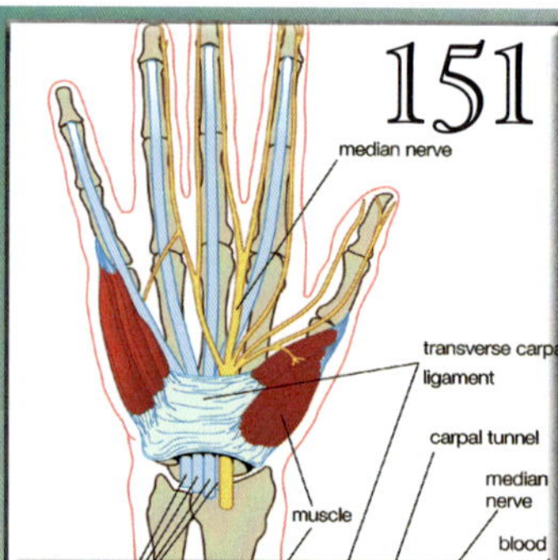
151
median nerve
ligament
carpal tunnel
median
nerve
muscle
blood

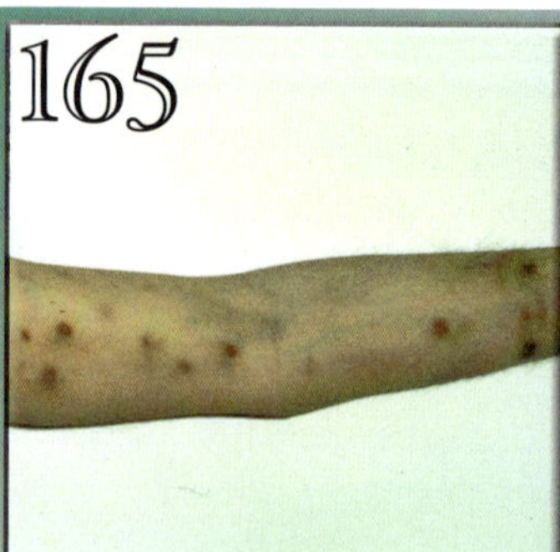
165

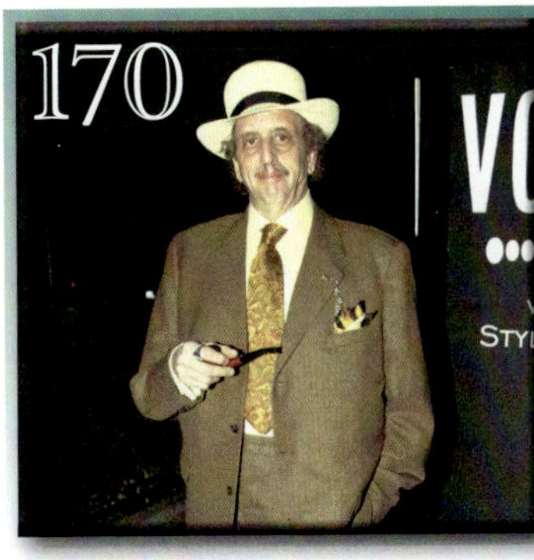
170

INTRODUCTION

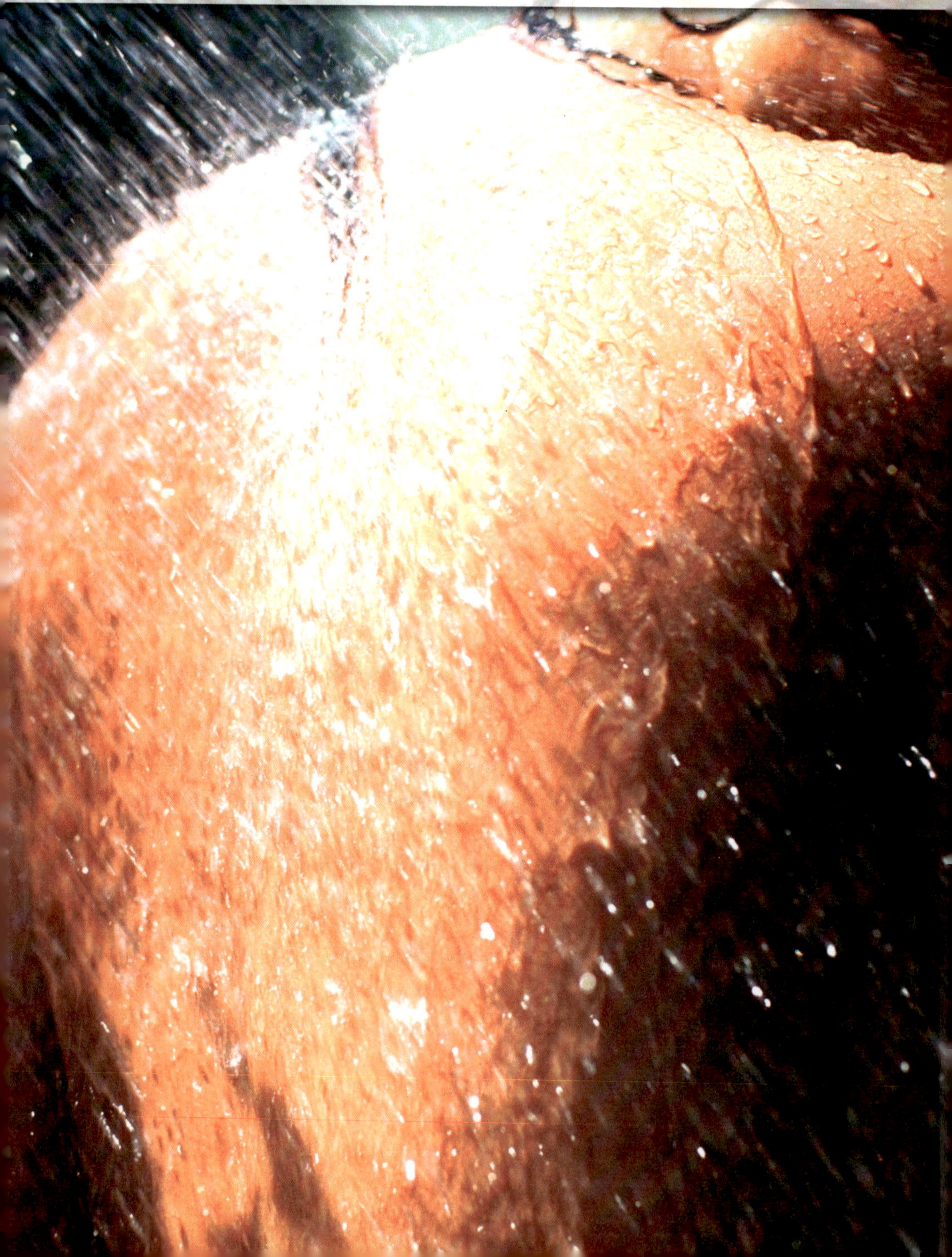

The human brain controls a person's actions and life functions, the heart pumps blood, and the lungs draw in oxygen that is transported through the blood stream to support bodily functions. But what about the skin and connective tissue? It is tempting to view skin as merely a casing, and connective tissue as the material that joins the bones of the skeleton together. Indeed, skin and connective tissue are the body's enclosure and binder, respectively. Yet they also protect and support internal organs, act as a line of defense against injury and disease, and give bodies the flexibility and sensitivity needed to survive. In this book, the structure and function of these amazing systems and the possible dysfunction and diseases that can beset them are examined thoroughly.

Skin serves two basic functions: to protect the body from the environment and help the body communicate with it. As a physical barrier, skin shields the body from Sun damage, injury, and germs. As a communicator, skin makes use of the cutaneous sense organs, or nerves. Nerves have different functions and abilities, according to their type, size, and location. So-called "free nerves" are located in the epidermis, the outermost portion of the skin, whereas corpuscular nerves are embedded in a deeper layer of the skin known as the dermis. Both types of nerves connect to the spine via a thick bundle of nerve fibres. The ability of nerves to transmit information regarding pressure, temperature, and pain enables humans to respond appropriately to various environmental stimuli.

Compared with that of other mammals, human skin has several unique features. For example, it is largely hairless, with the clusters of hair serving as social and sexual markers, as opposed to animal hair (fur) that is used primarily for warmth. Skin also has varying thicknesses on different parts of the human body, dictated by the need for flexibility, sensitivity, and strength.

Skin has many layers that crisscross over one another for structural and functional purposes. The outer layer, the epidermis, protects the body from illness by preventing many types of infectious organisms from entering the body. Pores in the skin act as a cooling system for the body, facilitating the release of sweat. Sweat also acts to keep the skin flexible, and even aids the ability to grip objects. A layer of keratin assists in holding epidermal cells together and prevents the escape of water from the body. In addition to skin cells, living and dead, the epidermis contains fine hairs, the follicles of which extend through the dermis, the underlying layer of skin. The dermis also contains nerves, blood and lymph vessels, and sebaceous and sweat glands.

Hair, though not necessarily needed for protection from the elements, provides sensory information to the brain. Hair follicles are surrounded by nerves, which relay vital information about touch to the brain. The sebaceous glands, also attached to the follicles, release sebum, a combination of fats and esters that appears to act as an emollient, keeping skin soft and supple. Blood vessels present in skin respond to the sensory information obtained from the surface, contracting and expanding to regulate blood flow and maintain body temperature and blood pressure. External factors such as pressure, heat, and muscle movement also affect the lymph vessels, which control the drainage of fluids.

Skin cells constantly renew themselves; the average life cycle of a skin cell is between one and three months. Cells multiply near the dermis layer and rise to the surface, producing keratin as they migrate through the epidermis. When the skin suffers a wound, cells multiply quickly; within 48 hours of injury, new skin begins to form.

The colour, or pigment, of a person's skin is due mainly to melanin. Produced by melanocytes in epidermal basal cells, melanin levels vary from person to person, although the number of melanocytes is roughly the same for each individual. Melanin also is found in hair, the eyes, and various internal membranes.

Connective tissue is the component that links the different parts of the body together and enables them to function as a unit. All connective tissue contains the same components, but it becomes specialized as one component becomes dominant. There are five specialized types of connective tissue in the human body: cartilage, ligaments, tendons, bones, and fat (or adipose) tissue.

Cartilage is rigid and resistant to compression, yet it is also able to grow. Bone is formed from cartilage in utero. There are three principal subtypes of cartilage: hyaline cartilage, located mainly on the surface of joints; elastic cartilage, which is present in the ears and throat; and fibrocartilage, found where tendons attach to bones and in spinal disks.

Ligaments support organs and connect bones at joints. There are two types of ligaments: white, which is high in collagen and inflexible, and yellow, which is made up of tough elastic fibres. Tendons act like bands that connect muscles to bones, transmitting force from the former to the latter.

Finally, bones are made up of calcified connective tissue, which gives structure to the body and provides a reserve of calcium that can be released as needed. Bones are coated with periosteum, a fibrous membrane that contains blood vessels, collagen, and osteoblasts, or bone-producing cells.

Connective tissue is composed mainly of various types of cells and fibres, including collagen, elastin, and reticular fibres. Collagen, the most abundant type of fibre, is present in varying levels in connective tissue. Also present in connective tissue is ground substance, a gel-like mix of carbohydrates and protein. Ground substance conveys material to and from tissue cells and also acts as a barrier to harmful substances, such as bacteria. Finally, two types of cells, stationary and migrating, are present in connective tissue. Stationary cells remain in a relatively fixed position. These include fibroblasts, which secrete tropocollagen to form scar tissue, and adipose cells, which synthesize and store nutrients. Migrating cells move freely through tissue to perform a variety of functions. One subcategory, mast cells, release histamines and heparin to widen blood vessels or prevent clotting. Another type of migrating cell, the monocyte, divides and moves to attack bacteria. In doing so, the monocyte cell dies and is secreted as pus.

In the womb, skin and connective tissue are formed from several different types of tissue. A fetus's ectoderm grows to become the epidermis and gives rise to hair and nails. Dermatome tissue also becomes skin and subcutaneous tissue, developing into those layers found primarily in the torso region. Human fetal skin cells undergo numerous transformations during their nine months of growth.

The skin is susceptible to a vast number of problems and malfunctions caused by external influences, illnesses, and even a person's emotions. Open wounds to the skin, such as cuts, expose the body to foreign elements, including bacteria and viruses. Blood rushes to the wound and dries to form a scab, which acts as a physical barrier to infection while bringing the edges of the cut skin together. After healing, scar tissue may be visible—the remnants of collagen fibres that have knit the wound together. Other force injuries to the skin include bruises, blisters, and calluses.

Frostbite is an injury to the skin caused by overexposure to cold temperatures. The dramatic loss of heat causes ice crystals to form in the fluids in the skin, damaging cells. Raising body temperature is the cure for frostbite, and quick action results in reduced permanent damage.

Skin infections occur when hostile foreign bodies penetrate the dermis. Regular cleansing of skin wounds helps prevent infection, and medications fight infections that are acquired. One common type of bacterial infection is impetigo, caused by infection with Streptococcus or Staphylococcus bacteria. Transmitted easily in hot, humid, and cramped environments, impetigo is common in children. It causes blisters that burst and scab over and may be treated with oral or topical antibiotics. Sometimes the site of a bacterial infection can become so badly damaged that an abscess forms. An abscess is a pocket of pus that accumulates in the cavity of a wound, the result of digestion of bacteria by white blood cells.

Fungal infections also can affect the skin. For instance, ringworm feeds on keratin and leaves circular scabs. Related to other common fungal infections, ringworm is treated with oral or topical antifungal medications. Other causes of skin infection include viruses, such as those that cause warts, and infestation by mites, which is the genesis of a highly communicable skin disease known as scabies.

Dermatitis, also known as eczema, comes in several forms. Contact dermatitis results from physical contact with a known allergic substance, such as poison ivy. Symptoms of dermatitis include reddened and flaking skin, swelling, and oozing blisters. Atopic dermatitis begins in infancy, and those afflicted frequently develop hay fever or asthma later in life, suggesting that immune function is a factor. A chronic type of skin inflammation, psoriasis is caused by a combination of environmental and genetic factors. Psoriasis is expressed in red, scaly papules on the skin and is treatable with medication, although it is incurable. A very common type of skin inflammation is sunburn. Caused by overexposure to ultraviolet (UV) light, sunburn is marked by symptoms, including redness, tenderness and swelling, that peak within the first two days after exposure. Preventative measures include avoiding peak sunlight hours and wearing sunscreen.

Connective tissue diseases generally are thought to be autoimmune in nature. Common clinical features of such diseases include joint inflammation, serous (fluid-exuding) membranes, and small blood vessels. Frequently, connective tissue dysfunction also involves various organs that have a high content of connective tissue, such as the lungs. One such disease, rheumatoid arthritis, is the chronic inflammation of the peripheral joints. Primarily affecting middle-aged women, rheumatoid arthritis begins in the tissue that lines the joints, eventually replacing it with scar tissue. This condition has a slow onset, starting with pain in the hands and feet; its outcome ranges from total recovery to partial paralysis.

Another connective tissue disease, polychondritis, affects cartilage. The inflammation associated with this condition ultimately destroys the cartilage in the middle ear, nose, and joints of afflicted individuals. While the disease is treatable, the damage it causes is irreversible.

Connective tissue is also subject to injury. Common disorders of overuse include tendinitis and carpal tunnel syndrome. Such conditions are treated with rest and external support or temporary immobilization of the affected area.

Skin and connective tissues also are susceptible to cancers and hereditary diseases. Melanoma, which is a cancer of melanocytes, accounts for roughly 5 percent of all cases of cancer diagnosed in the United States. The most serious and deadly form of skin cancer, melanoma is diagnosed by skin biopsy and is treated through a combination of surgery, chemotherapy, and radiation. Nonmelanoma skin cancers affect the surface tissue, and if detected early are far less likely to be fatal than melanomas. Avoidance of UV sunlight and frequent examination of moles for changes are preventative measures one can take to combat skin cancers of all types.

Connective tissue cancers, or sarcomas, are more likely to affect bone than soft tissue, and may be related to chromosomal abnormalities. Fibrosarcoma tumours typically grow in the bones of the thigh, upper arm, and jaw, but may affect surrounding tissues, making surgical removal difficult. Kaposi sarcoma is expressed through lesions on the skin and mucous membranes and is primarily found in individuals with HIV/AIDS.

Hereditary diseases of the skin and connective tissues often have severe outcomes. Several cause different types of skeletal deformity, such as achondroplasia, in which cartilage is unable to grow into bone; it is the chief cause of dwarfism. Intellectual disability is an affect of a class of hereditary diseases called mucopolysaccharidoses, which is characterized by the inability to properly metabolize carbohydrates in ground substance. Sanfilippo and Hurler syndromes are two examples of this type of disorder. Shortened life span is another consequence of some hereditary diseases of the skin and connective tissues.

Some diseases have localized symptoms. Dupuytren contracture, which is the thickening of the fascia in the palm, results in the permanent flexing of one or more fingers. Some diseases can weaken the body's structural elements, such as ostogenesis imperfecta, or brittle bone disease. Others create rigidity, as with myositis ossificans, in which connective tissue is replaced by bone over time.

Skin and connective tissue are complex components of the human body that are constantly changing and performing unseen functions. The intricacy and cooperative function of the two is a vast topic ripe for exploration.

CHAPTER 1

Anatomy of the Human Skin

The skin and connective tissue are vital components of the human body. Skin, which is the covering (or integument) of the body's surface, is the largest organ of the human body. It provides protection and receives sensory stimuli from the external environment. Connective tissue, on the other hand, provides a framework that supports the body's organs, including muscle and skin. By uniting muscles with tendons, ligaments, and bone, and by bringing elasticity to the skin, connective tissue enables the body to function as a cohesive unit, with the many parts moving together fluidly.

While connective tissue is made up of various combinations of cells, extracellular fibres, and a gel-like material known as ground substance, the skin consists of three well-defined layers of tissue: the epidermis, the dermis, and the subcutis. The epidermis is the outermost layer and contains the primary protective structure, the stratum corneum. The dermis is a fibrous layer lying beneath the epidermis that supports and strengthens the epidermis. The subcutis is a subcutaneous layer of fat that lies beneath the dermis, supplies nutrients to the other two layers, and cushions and insulates the body.

DISTINCTIVE FEATURES

The characteristic features of skin change from the time of birth to old age. In infants and children it is velvety, dry, soft, and largely free of wrinkles and blemishes.

Children younger than two years sweat poorly and irregularly, presumably because their sebaceous glands function minimally. At adolescence hair becomes longer, thicker, and more pigmented, particularly in the scalp, axillae, and pubic eminence, and on the male face. General skin pigmentation increases, localized pigmented foci appear mysteriously, and acne lesions often develop. Hair growth, sweating, and sebaceous secretions begin to blossom. As a person ages, anatomical and physiological alterations, as well as exposure to sunlight and wind, leave skin, particularly that not protected by clothing, dry, wrinkled, and flaccid.

Human skin, more than that of any other mammal, exhibits striking topographic differences. An example is

Cross Section of Human Skin

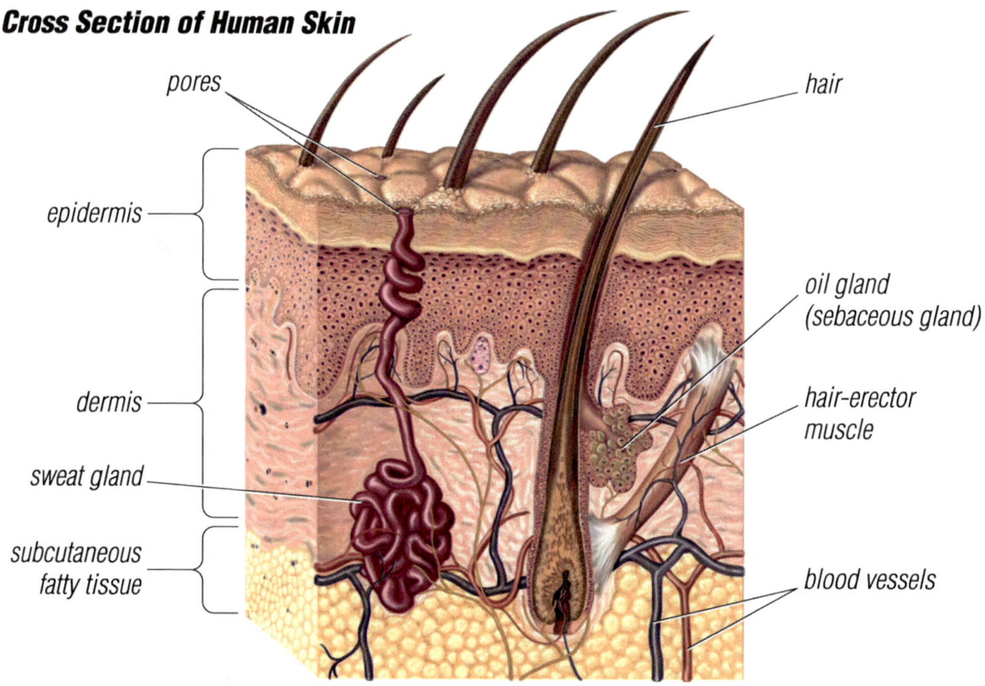

Section through human skin and underlying structures. Encyclopædia Britannica, Inc.

the dissimilarity between the palms and the backs of the hands and fingers. Likewise, whereas the skin of the eyebrows is thick, coarse, and hairy, that on the eyelids is thin, smooth, and covered with almost invisible hairs. The face is seldom visibly haired on the forehead and cheekbones. It is completely hairless in the vermilion border of the lips, yet coarsely hairy over the chin and jaws of males. The surfaces of the forehead, cheeks, and nose are normally oily, in contrast with the relatively greaseless lower surface of the chin and jaws. The skin of the chest, pubic region, scalp, axillae, abdomen, soles of the feet, and ends of the fingers varies as much structurally and functionally as it would if the skin in these different areas belonged to different animals.

The skin achieves strength and pliability by being composed of numbers of layers oriented so that each complements the others structurally and functionally. To allow communication with the environment, countless nerves—some modified as specialized receptor end organs and others more or less structureless—come as close as possible to the surface layer, and nearly every skin organ is enwrapped by skeins of fine sensory nerves.

THE DERMIS

The dermis makes up the bulk of the skin and provides physical protection. It is composed of an association of fibres, mainly collagen, with materials known as glycosaminoglycans, which are capable of holding a large amount of water, thus maintaining the turgidity of the skin. A network of extendable elastic fibres keeps the skin taut and restores it after it has been stretched.

The hair follicles and skin glands are derived from the epidermis but are deeply embedded in the dermis. The dermis is richly supplied with blood vessels, although none penetrates the living epidermis. The epidermis receives materials only by diffusion from below. The dermis also contains nerves and sense organs at various levels.

BLOOD AND LYMPH VESSELS

Human skin is enormously well supplied with blood vessels. It is pervaded with a tangled, though apparently orderly, mass of arteries, veins, and capillaries. Such a supply of blood, far in excess of the maximum biologic needs of the skin itself, is evidence that the skin is at the service of the blood vascular system, functioning as a cooling device. To aid in this function, sweat glands pour water upon its surface, the evaporation of which absorbs heat from the skin. If the environment is cold and body heat must be conserved, cutaneous blood vessels contract in quick, successive rhythms, allowing only a small amount of blood to flow through them. When the environment is warm, they contract at long intervals, providing a free flow of blood. During muscular exertion, when great quantities of generated heat must be dissipated, blood flow through the skin is maximal.

In addition to its control of body temperature, skin also plays a role in the regulation of blood pressure. Much of the flow of blood can be controlled by the opening and closing of certain sphincterlike vessels in the skin. These vessels allow the blood to circulate through the peripheral capillary beds or to bypass them by being shunted directly from small arteries to veins.

Human skin is permeated with an intricate mesh of lymph vessels. In the more superficial parts of the dermis, minute lymph vessels that appear to terminate in blind sacs function as affluents of a superficial lymphatic net that in turn opens into vessels that become progressively larger in the deeper portions of the dermis. The deeper, larger vessels are embedded in the loose connective tissue that surrounds the veins. The walls of lymph vessels are so flabby and collapsed that they often escape notice in specimens prepared for microscopic studies. Their abundance, however, has been demonstrated by injecting vital dyes inside the dermis and observing the clearance of the dye.

Because lymph vessels have minimal or no musculature in their walls, the circulation of lymph is sluggish and largely controlled by such extrinsic forces as pressure, skeletal muscle action, massaging, and heat. Any external pressure exerted, even from a fixed dressing, for example, interferes with its flow. Since skin plays a major role in immunologic responses of the body, its lymphatic drainage is as significant as its blood vascular system.

THE SKIN SURFACE

The intact surface of the skin is pitted by the orifices of sweat glands and hair follicles—the so-called pores—and is furrowed by intersecting lines that delineate characteristic patterns. All individuals have roughly similar markings on any one part of the body, but the details are unique. The lines are oriented in the general direction of elastic tension. Countless numbers of them, deep and shallow, together with the pores, give every region of the body a characteristic topography. Like the deeper furrows and ridges on the palms and soles, the skin lines are mostly established before birth. The fine details of each area of body surface are peculiar to each individual. Fingerprints are used as a means of personal identification because they have a high relief, more evident patternings, and can be easily obtained.

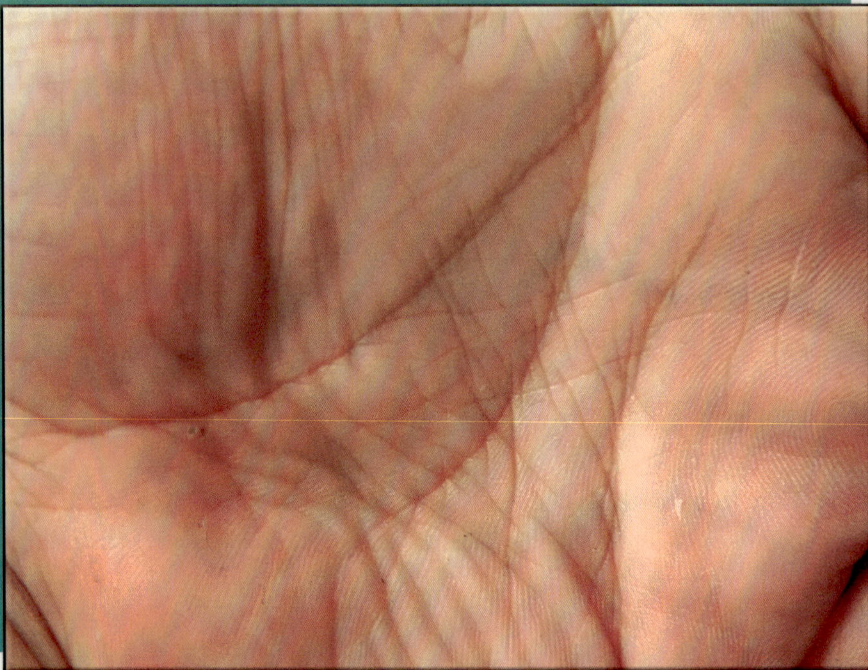

The lines on human palms start to form in utero, although they may be altered somewhat through use as a person ages. Shutterstock.com

Some of the lines on the surface of the skin are acquired after birth as a result of use or damage. For example, furrows on the forehead are an accentuation of preexisting congenital lines that become strongly emphasized in old age. As the skin becomes less firm with aging, it also forms wrinkles. Certain occupations leave skin marks that, depending upon duration and severity, may be transient or permanent.

The palms of the hands and the soles of the feet are etched by distinct alternating ridges and grooves that together constitute dermatoglyphics. The ridges follow variable courses, but their arrangement in specific areas has a consistent structural plan. Though apparently continuous, the ridges have many interruptions and irregularities, branching and varying in length. Every small area of surface has ridge details not matched anywhere in the same individual or in any other individual, even in an identical twin. This infallible signature makes dermatoglyphics the best-known physical characteristic for personal identification.

THE EPIDERMIS

The epidermis is thicker on the palms and soles than it is anywhere else and is usually thicker on dorsal than on ventral surfaces. Omitting the fine details, it is divisible everywhere into a lower layer of living cells and a superficial layer of compact dead cells.

General Structure

All the cells, living or dead, are attached to one another by a series of specialized surfaces called attachment plaques, or desmosomes. Thus, instead of being completely fused, the membranes of adjacent cells make a zipperlike contact, with fluid-filled spaces between the contact areas. This structural pattern ensures a concatenation of cells to one another so that they cannot be sloughed off easily. At the same time, this structure also allows nutrient fluids to seep in from the vessels in the dermis. Epidermal cells, which multiply chiefly at the base in contact with the dermis, gradually ascend to the surface, manufacturing keratin as they go. They finally die in the upper part, forming a horny layer.

The epidermis is thickest on friction surfaces and thinnest over the eyelids, on the lower parts of the abdomen, and around the external genitalia. Unlike that of most other mammals, it has an intricately sculptured underside and does not lie flat upon the dermis. Seen from beneath, there are straight and branching ridges and valleys, columns and pits, all finely punctuated.

Because of this unevenness, it is almost impossible to state the exact thickness of epidermal tissue. Furthermore, individual differences, sex, and age have an enormous influence on the structure of the underside. Such labyrinthine patterns give human epidermis two unique advantages: it attains a more intimate connection with the subjacent dermis than if the surface were flat, and its source of dividing cells, the building blocks of the horny layer, is greatly increased.

Major Layers

The clear stratification of the epidermis is the result of well-defined changes in its major constituent cells—the keratinocytes, or corneocytes—as they move peripherally from the basal layer, where they are continuously formed by mitosis, to the skin surface, where they are lost. In essence, the epidermis consists of a living malpighian layer (consisting of cells whose protoplasm has not yet changed into horny material), in contact with the basement membrane (which is attached to the dermis), and a superficial cornified (horny) layer of dead cells.

The innermost cells of the malpighian layer, next to the basement membrane, make up the basal layer, or *stratum basale*. Immediately peripheral to the basal layer is the spinous, or prickle-cell, layer—the stratum spinosum. Its cells have a spiny appearance due to the numerous desmosomes on their surface. Studies with the electron microscope have revealed that desmosomes are symmetrical, laminated structures in which some layers are contributed by the plasma membranes of adjoining cells and some form an intercellular component.

The spinous layer is succeeded by the granular layer, or stratum granulosum, with granules of keratohyalin contained in the cells. These small particles are of irregular shape and occur in random rows or lattices. The cells of the outer spinous and granular layers also contain much larger, lamellated bodies—the membrane-coating granules. They are most numerous within the cells of the spinous layer. In the granular layer they appear to migrate toward the periphery of each cell and to pass into the intercellular spaces, where they discharge their waxy lipid components.

Peripheral to the granular layer is the stratum corneum, or horny layer, in which the keratinocytes have lost their nuclei and most of their organelles and contents, including the keratohyalin granules. They become progressively flattened and filled with keratin and are ultimately desquamated. Between the granular layer and stratum corneum, an unstainable stratum lucidum, or hyaline layer, can be recognized in palmar and plantar epidermis and some other regions (palmar and plantar refer to the palm surface of the hand and the bottom surface of the foot, respectively).

Dynamics and Organization

Horizontal stratification is the most obvious histological feature of the epidermis. There is also, however, distinct evidence of vertical organization. In thin epidermis, though not in thick plantar skin, the cornified cells can be shown to be arranged in regular stacks, which must reflect the underlying dynamic mechanisms. It appears that several living spinous cells are precisely and symmetrically stacked beneath each cornified column and that these are related to their own basal cells. The cells do not pass from one stock to another.

All keratinocytes are formed by mitosis (cell division) in the lower region of the malpighian layer (the malpighian layer consists of both the stratum basale and the stratum spinosum of the epidermis). Most of the dividing cells are found in the basal layer, although it is likely that about one-third of the divisions occur above this level. Proliferating cells undergo a cycle: mitosis is followed by an interphase, this in turn is followed by a phase of DNA synthesis, and then another short resting phase occurs before mitosis begins again. The complete mitotic cycle takes about 12 to 19 days. The time for the passage of cells through the epidermis, from formation to desquamation, has been variously estimated at one to three months.

In normal skin the production and loss of cells must be finely balanced, otherwise the thickness of the epidermis would fluctuate. When the epidermis becomes abnormally thick, as in the plaques of psoriasis, this balance is altered. Either the production of cells in the malpighian layer must be abnormally high or their time of passage must be decreased. It is now generally agreed that such conditions result from a greatly increased production of cells, and the cells move more, not less, rapidly through the epidermis.

There is, however, a further controversial problem. If all the basal cells were continuously cycling, greater production could be achieved only by a substantial reduction in the duration of the cell cycle. An alternative hypothesis is that not all the cells are undergoing cycles at any one time, so that greater cell production can be achieved by recruiting resting cells into activity. It seems likely that the epidermis does indeed contain noncycling cells, which can become activated, and that the cell cycle in psoriatic epidermis is accelerated only about twofold, not twelvefold, as once proposed.

When skin is wounded, there is a burst of epidermal mitotic activity about 40 hours later. It is evident, therefore, that local mechanisms of control must come into play, with either inhibitors being dispersed by wounding, or stimulating hormones being released, or both. There is, on the one hand, some evidence of the existence of inhibitors, or chalones. On the other hand, an epidermal growth factor (EGF) has been isolated from the salivary glands of mice and its chemical structure determined (a single-chain, folded polypeptide with 53 amino acid residues and three intramolecular disulfide bonds). It is not, however, extractable from skin, though the receptor protein to which it attaches in order to perform its action is present in many skin cells, and a closely similar molecule has been isolated from human urine.

The Keratin Layer

The final product of the epidermis is the keratin that packs the cornified cells. The term *keratin* is applied generally to the hard keratins of hair, horn, and nails, and to the soft keratin of the epidermis. They are all insoluble filamentous proteins, composed of polypeptide chains that are stabilized by links using two atoms of sulfur. The source of the keratin of the stratum corneum has been a subject of controversy. However, it is now generally accepted that about a third of its total mass is made up of proteins synthesized in the granular layer and the remainder from so-called intermediate filaments, which are present in keratinocytes from the basal layer outward.

The barrier that prevents water loss from the body is situated in the lower part of the horny layer. In this region the spaces between the compacted layers of keratin-filled cells contain lamellae of lipid (wax) that has been formed within the membrane-coating granules of the live epidermal cells below.

Hair

The apparent lack of body hair immediately distinguishes humans from all other large land mammals. Regardless of individual or racial differences, the human body seems to be more or less hairless, in the sense that the hair is so vestigial as to seem absent. Yet, in certain areas hair grows profusely. These relatively hairy places may be referred to as epigamic areas, and they are concerned with social and sexual communication, either visually or by scent from glands associated with the hair follicles.

Human hair has little protective value, even in hirsute (excessively hairy) people. Eyelashes, eyebrows, and the hairs inside the external ears and nostrils have obviously useful functions, and scalp hair may be thick enough to provide some protection from the midday Sun. The beard and mustache, though, are embellishments, which establish maleness and are likely to be concerned with sexual or social communication. Axillary and pubic hair probably form part of scent-disseminating mechanisms.

An important role for hair, however, is its participation in the body's sensory apparatus. All hair follicles are surrounded by sensory nerves, and pressure on the hair shaft is transmitted to these nerves. Other mammals, including subhuman primates, have highly specialized sensitive hair follicles around the eyes, lips, and muzzle. These produce "tactile" hairs, known as vibrissae or

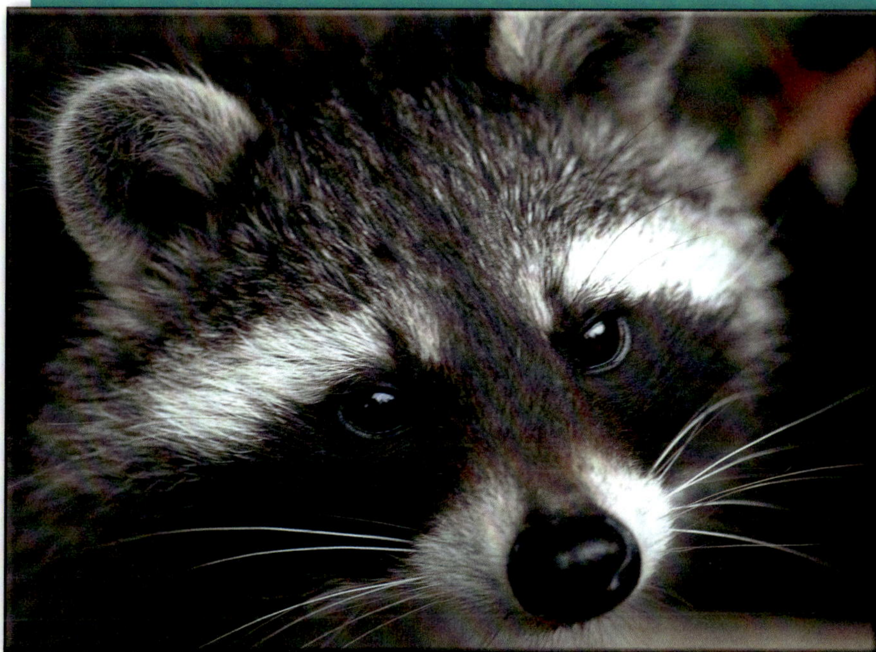

In addition to whiskers protruding from their muzzles, raccoons also have shorter vibrissae situated above their claws. Vibrissae help nocturnal animals like the raccoon maneuver and forage in the dark. Shutterstock.com

whiskers, which are particularly large in nocturnal mammals. The follicles from which these hairs emerge are rich in nerves and are surrounded by a sinus filled with blood. Humans are the only animals with no sinus hair follicles. Human hair follicles, however, particularly those of the face, are well supplied with nerves, and human skin is probably more sensitive than that of any other mammal.

Hairs are manufactured by follicles. Essentially, these are tubelike pockets of the epidermis that extend through most or all of the depth of the skin and enclose a small papilla of dermis in their base. They lie at an angle to the skin surface. Two-thirds of the way up is a bulge, and attached to it are wisps of smooth muscle fibre that, on contracting, pull the follicle to a more or less perpendicular position. This action also puckers the skin into a mound on the surface—a so-called goose pimple.

Exactly as in other mammals, the human hair is formed by division of cells in the region known as the bulb, at the base of the follicle. Pigment is incorporated from melanocytes in this region. Human hair follicles also go through cycles of activity. After a period of growth, the hair becomes clubbed, rather than cylindrical, in shape. Fibrous rootlets anchor the club to the surrounding follicular tissue. While forming the club, the follicle shrivels up, the lower part becoming largely dissipated. A resting follicle can be recognized at once by the clubbed hair and by the follicle's short size and unique structure. Follicles remain dormant for variable periods of time. When they become active again, they reconstruct a bulb that manufactures a new hair. As the new hair works its way to the surface, the club hair is loosened from its moorings and shed.

The activity of the hair follicles in the scalp is not synchronized, so that there is a small but steady molt of about 50 to 100 hairs a day from a total of around 150,000 follicles. There is, nevertheless, evidence of seasonal fluctuation, with the greatest hair loss in late summer and fall. A follicle may continue its activity for a long time, and hairs sometimes grow for several years and attain considerable lengths. Even in the human scalp—where the hair follicles are dense and vigorously productive—baldness occurs in a large number of individuals. Baldness is not a disease but is a systematic involution of hair follicles, culminating in organs similar to the primitive embryonic follicles. The numbers of follicles do not necessarily diminish.

Until late in fetal life there is no line of demarcation between the forehead and scalp. After the fifth month of gestation the follicles in the rest of the scalp grow larger, but those of the forehead do not. After birth the hairs on the forehead become even smaller and nearly invisible. The hairline of newborn infants is usually indistinct. The familial hairline pattern is defined late in childhood through a process that is identical with that of baldness. When male pattern baldness sets in, in the late 20s or earlier, the follicles affected undergo exactly the same changes as do those that establish the hairline.

Male pattern baldness and its female equivalent, which is usually more diffuse, are hereditary conditions. In males, this type of baldness is believed to arise from defects in the hair stem cells, which are located in the hair bulb and eventually mature into progenitor hair cells that then develop into mature hairs. Paradoxically, since male hormones (androgens) stimulate the growth of most other hair, this type of baldness occurs only if androgens are present.

Hairs vary in colour, diameter, and contour. The different colours result from variations in the amount, distribution, and type of melanin pigment in them, as well as from variations in surface structure that cause light to be reflected in different ways. Hairs may be coarse or so thin and colourless as to be nearly invisible. Straight hairs are round, while wavy hairs are alternately oval and round. Very curly and kinky hairs are shaped like twisted ribbons.

Human hair grows at the rate of about one-third of a millimetre a day, and once keratinized it is inert. If the colour or shape of a hair is altered as it is formed, several days must elapse before the effect becomes visible. Hairs become white with aging because of the failure of the melanocytes to inject pigment into the cells as they are formed. Tales of hair becoming white overnight may perhaps arise from cases of rapid differential shedding of pigmented hairs from a mixed population of white and dark ones, but the suggestion that individual dark hairs can somehow rapidly turn white is not true.

The beard and mustache are the most obvious examples of hair that requires male sex hormones, or androgens, for its growth. Facial hairs begin to develop at puberty, about two years after the start of pubic hair growth. The rate of growth of the beard initially increases with age, but levels out after 35. Hair on the chest—a traditional sign of masculinity—and that on the limbs are also androgen-dependent. Androgens cause longer hairs to be formed, partly by making them grow faster, but mainly by increasing the length of anagen, the growing phase. Fully formed hairs on the thigh are over three times longer in young men than in women, and the duration of anagen is around 54 days in males, compared with 22 days in females.

Pubic and axillary hair are also dependent on androgens, but they differ from other body hair in that they are luxuriant in females as well as in males. Their growth requires lower levels of hormone. The lower triangle of pubic hair is present in persons with a rare disease known as male pseudohermaphroditism. These individuals are genetic males who remain female in form until puberty because they lack an enzyme necessary to bind two atoms of hydrogen to the male hormone testosterone, which is responsible for male sex characteristics. Since persons with male pseudohermaphroditism lack facial hair, even when adults, it seems that beard growth requires the conversion of testosterone to dihydrotestosterone but that pubic hair growth does not.

Sebaceous Glands

The sebaceous glands are usually attached to hair follicles and pour their secretion, sebum, into the follicular canal.

In a few areas of the body, disproportionately large sebaceous glands are associated with very small hair follicles. In other areas, however, there are glands that are altogether free of follicles.

The outstanding feature of sebaceous glands is their holocrine mode of secretion, involving complete disintegration of the sebaceous cells. The glands consist of a series of lobes, or acini, each with a duct running toward the main sebaceous duct. The cells are generated by cell division around the periphery of each lobe. As they move toward the centre of the lobe and toward the duct, they synthesize and accumulate fat globules and become progressively larger and distorted. Ultimately they disintegrate to form the secretion.

Human sebum is a complex mixture of lipids—triglyceride fats (57.5 percent), wax esters (26 percent), squalene (12 percent), cholesterol esters (3 percent), and cholesterol (1.5 percent). The triglycerides are largely hydrolyzed by bacteria by the time the sebum reaches the skin surface, so that about a third of the surface fat consists of free fatty acids.

The activity of the sebaceous glands is mainly controlled by androgens. The glands are quite large at birth because of the influence of maternal hormones during development, but they regress soon afterward. They become active again at, or somewhat in advance of, the first signs of puberty. Their rate of secretion is a little higher in adult men than in women, and it falls off gradually with age in both sexes. It is very low in eunuchs (castrated males) but has been shown to increase when they are treated with androgens. That other factors—for example, pituitary hormones—may also influence secretion is suggested by the observation that sebum production is abnormally high in acromegaly, a disorder resulting from excessive secretion of growth hormone.

The function of sebum has been greatly debated. Some scientists have theorized that it is important as an emollient to prevent too rapid loss of water from the superficial layers of the stratum corneum. Others, however, have held that it is a functionless product of now useless, or vestigial, organs. Yet humans have more and larger glands than most mammals, and there is a specific plan in their distribution: they are largest and most numerous on the face and around the anogenital surfaces.

The skin around the nose, mouth, and forehead and over the cheekbones has beds of gigantic glands, the secretion of which keeps these surfaces constantly oily. The sebaceous glands evenly spaced in rows at the border of the eyelids—the meibomian glands—are so large that they are easily seen with the naked eye when the eyelids are everted (flipped inside-out). The glands on the genitalia produce copious amounts of sebaceous matter called smegma. Only humans have rich populations of sebaceous glands on the hairless surfaces of the lips. These glands increase in number and size as persons mature. The inside of the cheeks also has many large sebaceous glands, and occasionally there are glands even on the gums and tongue.

It seems highly unlikely, then, that sebum is functionless. While its significance is certainly not established, it is possible that it is concerned with subtle chemical communication by smell or taste. Such a function would bring humans into line with other mammals.

Sweat Glands

Sweat glands are coiled tubes of epidermal origin, though they lie in the dermis. Their secretory cells surround a central space, or lumen, into which the secretion is extruded. There are two distinct types: eccrine glands and apocrine glands. Eccrine glands open by a duct directly onto the skin surface, whereas apocrine glands usually develop in association with hair follicles and open into them.

Most other mammals have numerous apocrine glands in the hairy skin. Eccrine glands are usually absent from the hairy skin and limited to friction surfaces. In nonhuman primates there is a tendency for the number of eccrine sweat glands over the body to increase in progressively advanced animals at the same time that the number of apocrine glands becomes reduced. Prosimians (primitive primates, such as lemurs, lorises, and tarsiers) have only apocrine glands in the hairy skin. Eccrine glands begin to appear in some of the higher forms. The great apes either have equal numbers or have more eccrine than apocrine glands. Humans have the most eccrine glands, with apocrine glands restricted to specific areas.

Strictly speaking, apocrine glands have nothing to do with sweating. They appear late in fetal development (5 to 5½ months) nearly everywhere on the body. Most of these rudiments disappear within a few weeks except in the external ear canals, in the axillae, on the nipples of the breasts, around the navel, and on the anogenital surfaces. Single glands may be found anywhere. From this, one might speculate that the ancestors of humans had apocrine glands widely distributed over the body, and the embryonic rudiments may be reminders of the history of a once widespread organ system.

Where they appear, the apocrine glands are large and numerous. In the axilla they are so large that the coils press upon each other, forming adhesions and cross-shunts of such complexity that the glands are more spongy than tubular. The complex of these large apocrine glands commingled with an equal number of eccrine sweat glands in the axilla composes what is known as the axillary organ, one of the most characteristic features of human skin. Other than humans, only chimpanzees and gorillas have axillary organs. In spite of their large size, apocrine glands secrete only small amounts of a milky, viscid fluid—pale gray, whitish, yellow, or reddish—which contributes very little to axillary sweat. If eccrine glands were not there, the axillae would be relatively dry.

The odour of axillary secretion becomes more intense as it is decomposed by bacteria. Although axillary odours frequently seem unpleasant, they are not invariably so. The odour of individual humans comes mostly from apocrine secretion, with some contribution from sebum. Since the body odours of all other animals have a social or sexual significance, it can be assumed that this is the archetypal purpose of apocrine secretion, even in humans. The view that the axillary organs are scent glands is supported by the finding that androsterones—the compounds that are responsible for the odour of the boar to which the sow responds—also occur in human axillary secretions.

Humans have 2,000,000 to 5,000,000 eccrine sweat glands, with an average distribution of 150 to 340 per square centimetre. They are most numerous on the palms and soles and then, in decreasing order, on the head, trunk, and extremities. Some individuals have more glands than others, but there is no difference in number between men and women.

The specific function of sweat glands is to secrete water upon the surface so that it can cool the skin when it evaporates. The purpose of the glands on the palms and soles, however, is to keep these surfaces damp, to prevent flaking or hardening of the horny layer, and thus to maintain tactile sensibility. A dry hand does not grip well and is minimally sensitive.

The eccrine glands, then, can be divided into those that respond to thermal stimulation, the function of which is thermoregulation, and those that respond to psychological stimuli and keep friction surfaces moist. This makes a clear-cut distinction between the glands on the hairy surfaces and those on the palms and soles. In addition to thermal and psychological sweating, some individuals sweat on the face and forehead in response to certain chemical substances.

The glands on the palms and soles develop at about 3½ months of gestation, whereas those in the hairy skin are the last skin organs to take shape, appearing at 5 to 5½ months, when all the other structures are already formed. This separation of events over time may represent a fundamental difference in the evolutionary history of the two types of glands. Those on palms and soles, which appear first and are present in all but the hooved mammals, may be more ancient. Those in the hairy skin, which respond to thermal stimuli, may be more recent organs.

The sweat glands in the hairy skin of subhuman primates possibly function subliminally, although they are structurally similar to those of humans. The skin of monkeys and apes remains dry even in a hot environment. Profuse thermal sweating in humans, then, seems to be a new function. Eccrine sweat glands respond to a variety of drugs with different properties. They often respond differently in different individuals under nearly identical conditions and sometimes even respond inconsistently in the same individual. Notwithstanding these apparent vagaries, the eccrine glands function continuously, although their secretion may be imperceptible. Sweating is essential for keeping the human body from becoming overheated.

Nails

A major characteristic of primates is that their fingers and toes terminate in nails rather than in claws. One can speculate that the development of nails into flattened plates reflects the discontinuation of their use for digging or for defending and attacking. In a broad sense, nails are analogous to hair, having similar composition (keratin) and some common structural features. Even their genesis and mode of growth are comparable, but not identical, to those of hair.

Although apparently simple structures, nails are formed by complex and still poorly understood structural entities referred to as nail organs. Unlike hair, nails grow continuously, with no normal periods of rest. If their free edges were protected from wear, they would extend to prodigious lengths, growing in a twisted fashion like a ram's horns. Nails grow about 0.1 millimetre per day, or roughly one-third as rapidly as hair. Growth is somewhat slower in winter than in summer and slower in infants and old people than in vigorous young adults. It requires about three months for a whole nail to replace itself.

A number of factors can alter normal nail growth, among them age, trauma, poisons, and organic disorders. Habitual nail biting speeds up growth, and certain occupational practices can cause an increase in thickness. The nail-forming organ is particularly sensitive to physiological changes. During stressful periods or prolonged fever, or in response to noxious drugs, nails may become cracked, thinner, thicker, furrowed, or otherwise deformed, or they may be shed. Such sensitivity of response should make nails relatively good indexes of the health of individuals. But because of their ready response to so many internal and external factors, and because changes in them often

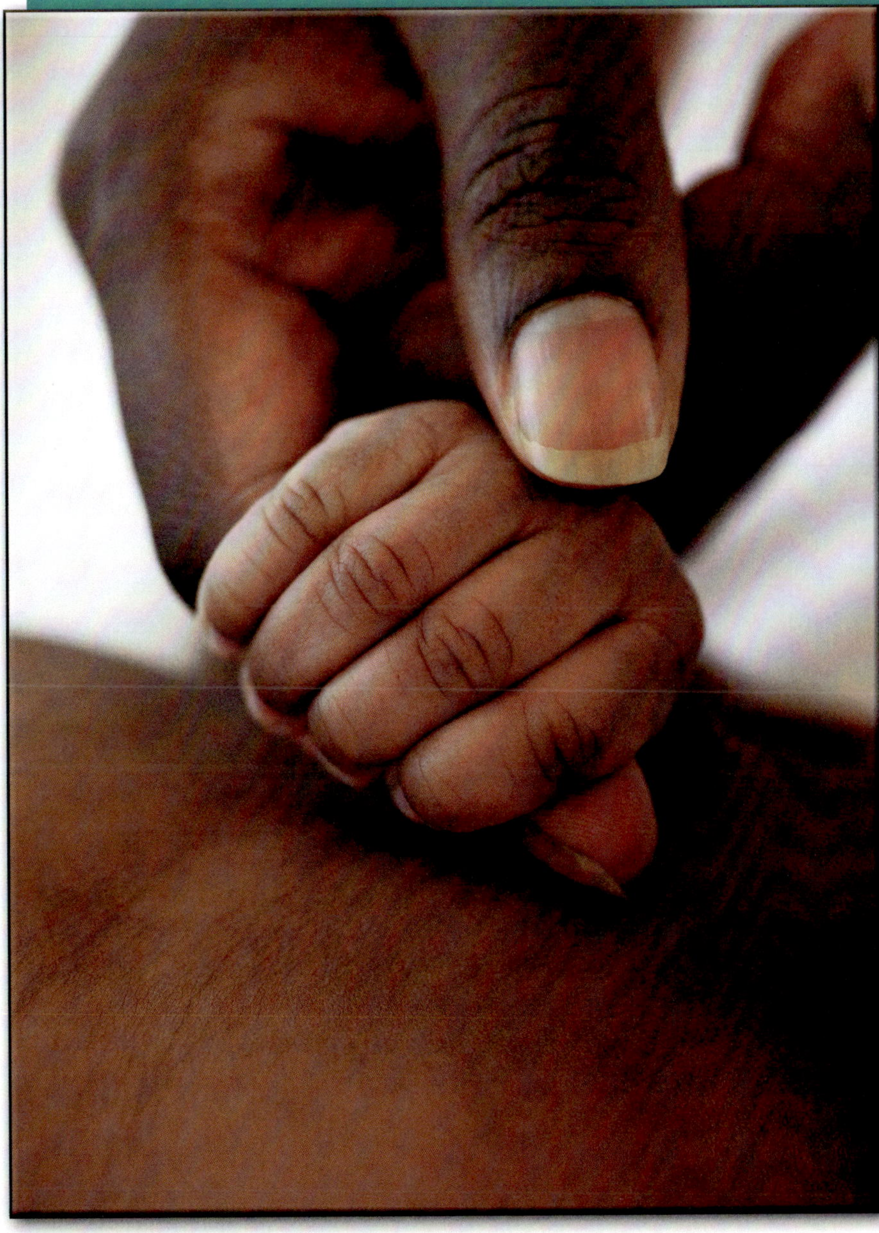

The term "lunule," describing the whitish arch at the base of a person's nails, comes from "lunar," meaning "moon." The lunule has a shape similar to a half or crescent moon. Shutterstock.com

occur without a known reason, signs of abnormality can be misleading or difficult to interpret. Like hair, the visible part of the nail plate is a dead structure. Defects inflicted upon it by mechanical means that do not disturb the underlying living tissue are eventually cast off at the free border.

Nails have a root, buried beneath the skin; a plate that is firmly attached to a nail bed underneath; and a free edge. Depending upon its thickness and the quality of its surface, the nail plate may be pink or whitish. The nail itself is translucent and colourless, allowing the colour of the blood in the superficial capillaries of the nail bed to show through. At its base the nail plate may have a whitish, arched marking called a lunule. Always present on thumbnails, lunules may be present or absent on the other fingers and are nearly always absent on the little finger. There are variations in different individuals and even between the two hands of the same person; such variations are probably controlled by genetic factors.

The nail itself consists of firmly cemented keratinized cells, flattened horizontally to the surface. Whereas the surface of nail plates may appear to be smooth, it is lined by parallel, longitudinal furrows, more strongly etched in some persons than in others and typically more prominent in the aged. These markings have some correspondence to the more pronounced grooves and ridges on the undersurface of the plate.

Nails grow from a matrix at the base of the nail root. During the early part of their journey, matrix cells multiply and move forward, synthesizing keratin, underneath the fold of skin (eponychium) at the base of the nail. Once exposed to the surface, the nail is fully formed. The nail plate seems to glide over the nail bed, but it is firmly attached to it. The entire tissue, nail bed and plate, most likely moves forward as a unit. The nail bed has often been called sterile matrix, since it adds little or nothing to the nail plate. Yet under certain pathologic conditions, it assumes keratinizing activities that result in a variably thickened or deformed nail plate.

Although less effective than claws for digging or gouging, the flattened nail is still an excellent adaptation that has added much to the development of manipulative skills. Nails not only protect the tips of fingers but also give them firmness and the ability to pick up or make contact with minute objects. Claws would be useless for such functions.

CHAPTER 2

CHARACTERISTICS OF CONNECTIVE TISSUE

Connective tissue maintains the form of the body and its organs and provides cohesion and internal support. The connective tissues include several types of fibrous tissue that vary only in their density and cellularity, as well as the more specialized and recognizable variants—bone, ligaments, tendons, cartilage, and adipose (fat) tissue.

While some organs are suspended from the wall of a body cavity by thin sheets of connective tissue called mesenteries, others are embedded in adipose tissue, a form of connective tissue in which the cells are specialized for the synthesis and storage of energy-rich reserves of fat, or lipid. The entire body is supported from within by a skeleton composed of bone, a type of connective tissue endowed with great resistance to stress owing to its highly ordered laminated structure and to its hardness, which results from deposition of mineral salts in its fibres and amorphous matrix. The individual bones of the skeleton are held firmly together by ligaments, and muscles are attached to bone by tendons, both of which are examples of dense connective tissue in which many fibre bundles are associated in parallel array to provide great tensile strength. At joints, the articular surfaces of the bones are covered with cartilage, a connective tissue with an abundant intercellular substance that gives it a firm consistency well adapted to permitting smooth gliding movements between the apposed surfaces. The synovial membrane, which lines the margins of the joint cavity

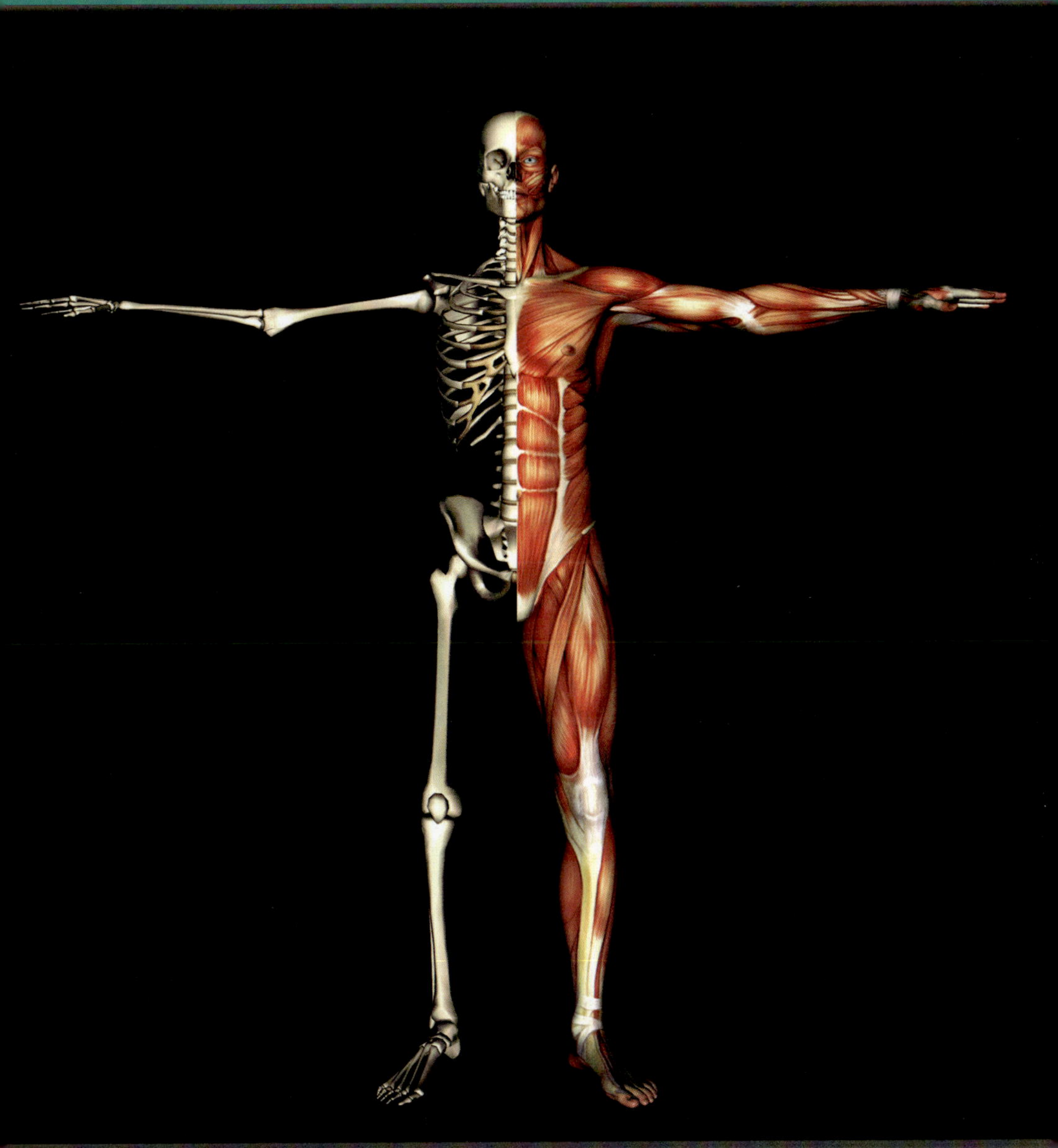

Human bones and muscles are held together by bundles of connective tissue called ligaments and tendons, respectively. Bones themselves are a strong, fortified laminate of connective tissue. Shutterstock.com

and lubricates and nourishes the joint surfaces, is also a form of connective tissue.

Blood vessels, both large and small, course through connective tissue, which is therefore closely associated with the nourishment of tissues and organs throughout the body. All nutrient materials and waste products exchanged between the organs and the blood must traverse perivascular spaces occupied by connective tissue. One of the important functions of the connective-tissue cells is to maintain conditions in the extracellular spaces that favour this exchange.

COMPONENTS OF CONNECTIVE TISSUE

All forms of connective tissue are composed of (1) extracellular fibres, (2) an amorphous matrix called ground substance, and (3) stationary and migrating cells. The proportions of these components vary from one part of the body to another depending on the local structural requirements. In some areas, the connective tissue is loosely organized and highly cellular. In other areas, its fibrous components predominate, and in still others, the ground substance may be its most conspicuous feature. The anatomical classification of the various types of connective tissue is based largely upon the relative abundance and arrangement of these components.

Extracellular Fibres

The fibrous components are of three kinds: collagenous, elastic, and reticular. Most abundant are the fibres composed of the protein collagen. The fibrous components of loose areolar connective tissue, when viewed with the light microscope, appear as colourless strands of varying diameter running in all directions, and, if not under tension, these have a slightly undulant course. At high magnification, the larger strands are seen to be made up of bundles of smaller fibres. The smallest fibres visible with the light microscope can be shown with the electron microscope to be composed of multiple fibrils up to 1000 angstroms (one Å = 1×10^{-7} mm) in diameter. These unit fibrils are cross-striated with transverse bands repeating every 640 Å along their length.

Collagen is of commercial as well as medical interest. Leather is the dense collagen of the dermis of animal skins preserved and toughened by the process called tanning. Fresh collagen dissolves in hot water, and the product is gelatin.

Under appropriate conditions, collagen can be brought into solution without chemical change. The fundamental units in such solutions are slender tropocollagen molecules about 14 Å wide and 2800 Å long. Collagen appears to be secreted in this form by the connective-tissue cells called fibrocytes, and the tropocollagen molecules assemble extracellularly to form striated collagen fibrils. By an alteration of the physicochemical conditions, tropocollagen in solution can be induced to polymerize with the formation of cross-striated fibrils identical to native collagen, thus simulating in the test tube the process of assembly that is believed to take place during fibrogenesis in the living organism. Analysis of the structure of collagen by X-ray diffraction has shown that the tropocollagen molecule consists of three side-by-side polypeptide chains—linear combinations of a number of amino acids, which are subunits of proteins—each in the form of a left-handed helix. These three left-handed helices are further twisted around one another to form a major right-handed helix.

Upon chemical analysis, the amino acid composition of collagen is found to be unique in its high proline content and in the fact that one-third of the amino acid residues are glycine. It is the only naturally occurring protein known to contain significant amounts of both hydroxyproline and hydroxylysine. Two of the three polypeptide chains comprising the tropocollagen molecule are similar in amino acid composition, while the third is distinctly different. In the tissues, the collagen fibrils are believed to be held together by a polysaccharide component.

Collagen is made up of about 15 percent proline. Proline is unique in that it contains a secondary amino group (-NH) rather than the primary amino group ($-NH_2$) characteristic of most amino acids. In addition, unlike other amino acids, proline, first isolated from casein (1901), is readily soluble in alcohol. Proline is one of several so-called nonessential amino acids (i.e., animals can synthesize it from glutamic acid and do not require dietary sources). The chemical structure of proline is

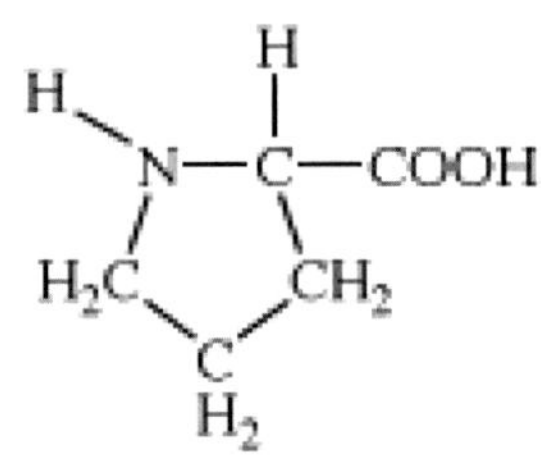

proline
(Pro, P)

Hydroxyproline constitutes about 14 percent of the amino acid content of collagen. First isolated (1902) from gelatin, a breakdown product of collagen, hydroxyproline, like proline, is a nonessential amino acid. Excretion of abnormal quantities of hydroxyproline is a symptom of the connective-tissue disease called Marfan syndrome. Also similar to proline, the molecular structure of hydroxyproline contains a secondary amino group (-NH) rather than the primary amino group (-NH_2). Its structure is:

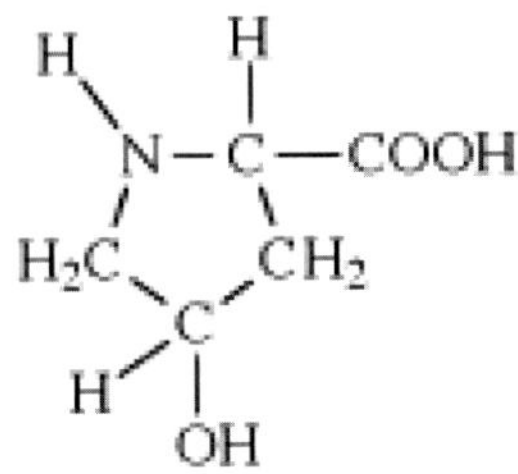

hydroxyproline (Hypro)

The hydroxylysine component of collagen is believed to play an important role in stabilizing intramolecular and intermolecular cross-links in collagen. This cross-linking capacity appears to be a function of the hydroxyl groups (-OH) present on hydroxylysine. These groups also serve as attachment sites for carbohydrates, particularly certain forms of galactose and glucosylgalactose. The attachment of these carbohydrates occurs via a process known as glycosylation. The purpose of hydroxylysine glycosylation is unclear, although it may play a role in dictating the organization of collagen fibres.

Elastic fibres are composed of the protein elastin and differ from collagenous fibres in dimensions, pattern, and chemical composition. They do not have uniform subunits comparable to the unit fibrils of collagen. They present a variable appearance in electron micrographs. Sometimes they appear to have an amorphous core surrounded by minute fibrils, while in other sites they appear to consist exclusively of dense amorphous material. Whether there are in fact two components or whether these are differing forms of the same substance is not yet clear.

At the light-microscope level, elastic fibres vary in diameter and often branch and reunite to form extensive networks in loose connective tissue. When present in high concentration, they impart a yellow colour to the tissue. In elastic ligaments, the fibres are very coarse and are arranged in parallel bundles. In the walls of arteries, elastin is present in the form of sheets or membranes perforated by openings of varying size. Elastic fibres are extremely resistant to hot water, to strong alkali, and even to digestion with the proteolytic enzyme trypsin. They can be digested, however, by a specific enzyme, elastase, present in the pancreas. Upon chemical analysis, elastin, like collagen, is found to be rich in glycine and proline, but it differs in its high content of valine and in the presence of an unusual amino acid, desmosine. As their name implies, elastic fibres are highly distensible and, when broken, recoil like rubber bands. Changes in this property and diminution in their numbers are thought to be, in part, responsible for the loss of elasticity of the skin and of the blood-vessel walls in old age.

Reticular fibres are distinguished by their tendency to form fine-meshed networks around cells and cell groups and by virtue of their property of staining black, because of adsorption of metallic silver, when they are treated with alkaline solutions of reducible silver salts. They were formerly believed to be composed of a distinct protein, reticulin, but electron microscopy has revealed that reticular fibres are small fascicles of typical collagen fibrils interwoven to form a network. It is now apparent that reticular fibres are simply a form of collagen, and their distinctive staining depends upon the mode of association of the fibrils and possibly upon subtle differences in their relation to the polysaccharide material that binds them together.

Ground Substance

The amorphous ground substance of connective tissue is a transparent material with the properties of a viscous solution or a highly hydrated thin gel. Its principal constituents are large carbohydrate molecules or complexes of protein and carbohydrate, called glycosaminoglycans (also known as mucopolysaccharides). One of these carbohydrates is hyaluronic acid, composed of glucuronic acid and an amino sugar, *N*-acetyl glucosamine. Other carbohydrates of the connective tissue are chondroitin-4-sulfate (chondroitin sulfate A) and chondroitin-6-sulfate (chondroitin sulfate C). The sugars of the sulfates are galactosamine and glucuronate.

Multiple chains of chondroitin sulfate seem to be bound to protein. These substances in solution are viscous. All substances passing to and from cells must pass through the ground substance. Variations in its composition and viscosity may therefore have an important influence on the exchange of materials between tissue cells and the blood. Its physical consistency also constitutes a barrier to the spread of particulates introduced into the tissues. It is interesting, in this relation, that some bacteria produce an enzyme, hyaluronidase, which breaks up hyaluronic acid into subunits and alters the viscosity of ground substance. The ability of these bacteria to produce this enzyme is probably responsible for their invasiveness in the tissues.

Cells of Connective Tissue

The cells of connective tissue include two types that are relatively stationary—fibrocytes and adipose cells—and several types of motile migrating cells—mast cells, macrophages, monocytes, lymphocytes, plasma cells, and eosinophils.

All the cells of connective tissue develop during embryonic life from the mesenchyme, a network of primitive stellate cells that have the potential for differentiating along several different lines depending upon local conditions. In addition to the specialized cell types of adult connective tissue described in the following pages, it is believed that small numbers of mesenchymal cells (stem cells) persist into postnatal life in the walls of small blood vessels and elsewhere and that these retain the capacity to differentiate into fibrocytes, adipose cells, macrophages, or a multitude of other cell types as the need arises.

Stationary Cells

The ubiquitous fibroblasts are the principal active cells of connective tissue, occurring as long spindle-shaped cells stretched along bundles of collagen fibrils. Their function is to secrete tropocollagen and constituents of the ground substance and to maintain these extracellular tissue components. When organs are injured, it is believed that cells known as fibrocytes, which reside in the stroma, are stimulated to develop into fibroblasts. The fibroblasts then migrate into the defect and deposit an abundance of new collagen, which forms a fibrous scar.

Adipose, or fat, cells are connective-tissue cells that are specialized for the synthesis and storage of reserve nutrients. Adipose cells may occur in small numbers anywhere in connective tissue, but they tend to develop preferentially along the course of small blood vessels.

There are two types of adipose cells: white adipose cells and brown adipose cells. White adipose cells contain large fat droplets, only a small amount of cytoplasm, and flattened, noncentrally located nuclei. Brown adipose cells, on the other hand, contain fat droplets of differing size, a large amount of cytoplasm, numerous mitochondria, and round, centrally located nuclei. The chief chemical constituents of adipose cell fat are triglycerides, which are esters made up of a glycerol and one or more fatty acids, such as stearic, oleic, or palmitic acids. Enzymes contained in adipose cells specialize in the hydrolysis of triglycerides in order to generate fatty acids and glycerol for physiological processes. The fat stored in these cells in part comes directly from the fats eaten and in part is manufactured within the body from fats and carbohydrates in the food and sometimes from protein. The main reservoir of fat in the body is the adipose tissue beneath the skin, called the panniculus adiposus.

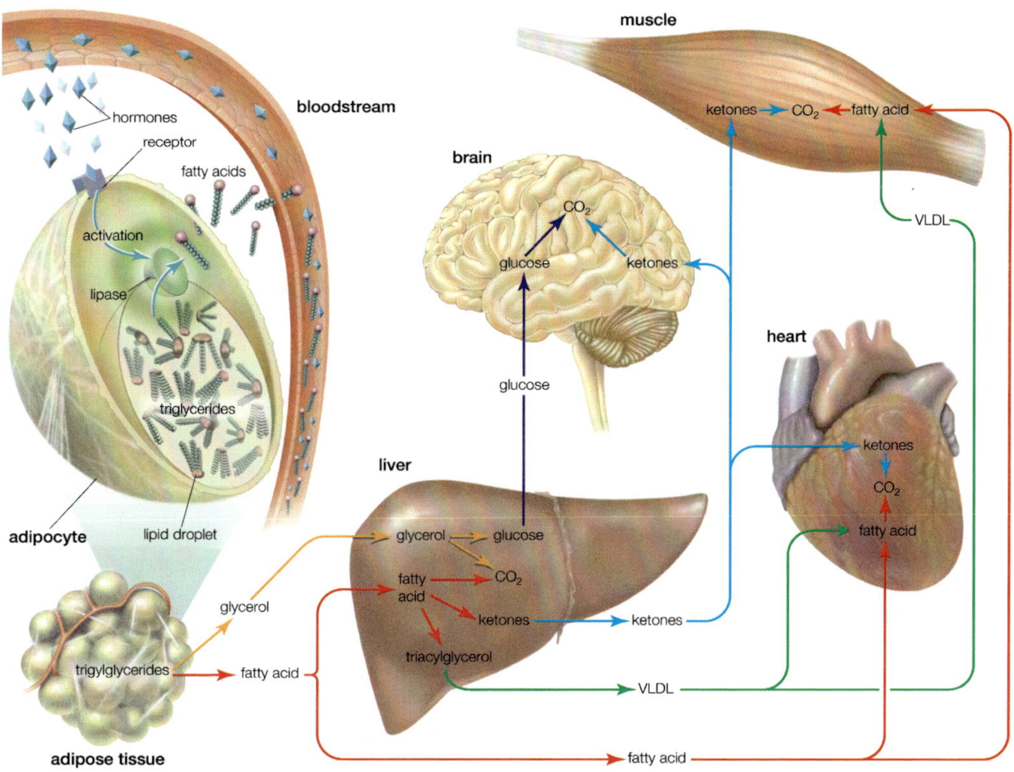

When hormones signal the need for energy, fatty acids and glycerol are released from triglycerides stored in fat cells (adipocytes) and are delivered to organs and tissues in the body. Encyclopædia Britannica, Inc.

There are also deposits of fat between the muscles, among the intestines and in their mesentery, around the heart, and elsewhere. One function of these deposits is to act as soft, elastic padding between the various organs.

Adipose tissue, which is in part made up of adipose cells, acts as a fuel reserve and helps conserve the heat of the body. In times of significant energy expenditure (e.g., exercise) or lack of adequate energy intake (e.g., fasting), adipose cells secrete fatty acids, which can be used by muscles and other tissues as a source of energy. Fatty acids generated by brown adipose cells generally are not secreted; instead, they are used by the cells' mitochondria in order to generate heat (thermogenesis), particularly in hibernating animals and human infants. Adipose cells also synthesize and secrete complex fatty acid substances called prostanoids (e.g., prostaglandins), which have various hormonelike actions such as inhibiting the breakdown of fat, and a protein hormone called leptin, which plays a role in the regulation of metabolism, body weight, and reproductive function. Adipose cells also express receptors capable of binding specific steroid hormones that can signal for increased storage of fat or increased release of fatty acids. Substances secreted but not synthesized by adipose cells include cholesterol and retinol (vitamin A).

Studies have shown that when old adipose cells die they are replaced by new cells and that in adult humans the number of adipose cells in the body is relatively stable. As a result, fat storage is accomplished through the expansion of existing adipose cells instead of through an increase in the number of cells. Likewise, when fat is utilized by the body, adipose cells shrink in size, as opposed to decreasing in number. The amount of fat contained in adipose cells can have significant effects on overall health. For example, too little fat can lead to reproductive dysfunction (e.g., amenorrhea in women), whereas excess fat can lead to obesity, cardiovascular disease, cancer, or diabetes. There also exist a group of rare genetic disorders known as lipodystrophies, which are characterized by the partial or complete absence of adipose tissue and may be acquired or inherited.

Because brown adipose cells function primarily as energy consumers and white adipose cells function primarily as energy stores, the common origin of these cells has been debated. In general, brown and white adipose cells are not found together; they form distinct tissues. Research has shown that brown adipose cells and muscle cells originate from the same precursor cells. The precursor cells are directed toward development into brown adipose cells by a specific protein, and, in the absence of this protein cue, the precursor cells become muscle cells. In addition, undifferentiated brown adipose cells contain ribonucleic acid (RNA) molecules that are similar to the RNA molecules of muscle cells. However, the RNA molecules in brown adipose cells disappear as the cells differentiate. In contrast, white adipose cells do not arise from the precursors of brown adipose cells and do not have any features of muscle cells. The discovery of the presence of brown adipose tissue in some adult humans indicates that insight into the mechanisms underlying brown adipose cell development may have implications in the treatment of obesity.

Migrating Cells

In addition to the relatively fixed cell types, there are free cells that reside in the interstices of loose connective tissue. These vary in their abundance and are free to migrate through the extracellular spaces. Among these wandering cells are the mast cells. Mast cells have a cell body filled with coarse granules that contain two biologically active substances, histamine and heparin. Histamine affects vascular permeability, and heparin, when added to blood, delays or prevents its clotting. Mast cells respond to mechanical or chemical irritation by discharging varying numbers of their granules. Histamine released from them causes fluid to escape from neighbouring capillaries or venules. This results in local swelling, as seen in the welt that appears around an insect bite.

Eosinophils are a type of white blood cell, or leukocyte. Some of these migrate through the walls of capillaries and take up residence in the connective tissues. They have polymorphous nuclei and, in the cell substance outside the nuclei, coarse granules that stain with eosin and other acid dyes. In electron micrographs, the granules contain conspicuous crystals. The granules have been isolated and shown to contain a variety of hydrolytic enzymes. Eosinophils are normally widespread in connective tissues of the body, but they are especially abundant in persons suffering from allergic diseases. The cells are believed to phagocytose and break down antigen-antibody complexes.

Plasma cells are mature antibody-secreting lymphocytes that are present in limited numbers in loose connective tissues and in larger numbers in lymphoid tissue. Lymphocytes are a type of leukoctye that is able to recognize foreign proteins and to respond to their presence by proliferating and differentiating into plasma cells. The plasma cells in turn synthesize and release specific immunoglobulins, called antibodies, that combine with and neutralize the foreign proteins. Lymphocytes are among the normal cellular elements of the blood, but they may also leave the blood and migrate in the connective tissues. They constitute an important reserve of relatively undifferentiated cells capable of sustaining an immunological response.

Another of the leukocytes that enter the connective tissues from the blood is the monocyte, a mononuclear cell larger than the lymphocyte and with different potentialities. These migratory cells can divide and, when appropriately stimulated, can transform into highly phagocytic macrophages. The reaction of the blood and connective-tissue cells to injury is called inflammation and is usually accompanied by local heat, swelling, redness, and pain. Under these conditions, the neutrophilic leukocytes (white blood cells called neutrophilic because of their neutral staining characteristics with certain dyes), which are not normally present in connective tissue in significant numbers, may migrate through the capillary walls in astronomical numbers and join the macrophages in the work of ingesting and destroying bacteria. Voraciously phagocytic, the neutrophils have a short life span. After having accomplished their mission, they die in great numbers. Pus, which may accumulate at sites of acute inflammation, is composed largely of dead and dying neutrophilic leukocytes.

The macrophages, or histiocytes, are derived from circulating monocytes in the bloodstream. They are also important for tissue repair and for defense against bacterial invasion. They have a great capacity for phagocytosis—the process by which cells engulf cellular debris, bacteria, or other foreign matter and break them down by intracellular digestion. Thus, they represent an important force of mobile scavenger cells.

TYPES OF CONNECTIVE TISSUE

The description presented thus far applies to the widely distributed loose areolar connective tissue, which is relatively unspecialized and can therefore be considered prototypic. In the more specialized forms of connective tissues, one component or another may predominate over all the others, depending upon the local structural or metabolic requirements. Adipose tissue, for example, is a variant of loose areolar tissue in which large numbers of adipose cells make up the bulk of the tissue.

Dense fibrous connective tissue is composed of closely packed bundles of collagen and their associated fibroblasts, but there are relatively few elastic fibres and little ground substance. The term *irregular dense fibrous tissue* is applied to sites where the collagen bundles are randomly oriented and interwoven, as in the dermis of the skin and the capsules of joints. *Regular dense fibrous tissue* is the term used to describe tendons, ligaments, and aponeuroses (fibrous sheets that form attachments for muscles), where the collagen fibres are precisely oriented in parallel bundles.

The synovial membrane, which lines joint capsules, is composed of loose vascular connective tissue but has cells specialized for secretion of the viscous synovial fluid, which is rich in hyaluronic acid, and for phagocytic functions. This fluid serves as a lubricant and nutrient for the avascular joint surfaces. Similar tissue forms sheaths around tendons where they pass over bony prominences.

Cartilage

Cartilage is a form of connective tissue in which the ground substance is abundant and of a firmly gelated consistency that endows this tissue with unusual rigidity and resistance to compression. The cells of cartilage, called chondrocytes, are isolated in small lacunae within the matrix. Although cartilage is avascular, gaseous metabolites and nutrients can diffuse through the aqueous phase of the gel-like matrix to reach the cells. Cartilage is enclosed by the perichondrium, a dense fibrous layer lined by cells that have the capacity to secrete hyaline matrix.

Cartilage grows by formation of additional matrix and incorporation of new cells from the inner chondrogenic layer of the perichondrium. In addition, the young chondrocytes retain the capacity to divide even after they become isolated in lacunae within the matrix. The daughter cells of these divisions secrete new matrix between them and move apart in separate lacunae. The capacity of cartilage for both appositional and interstitial growth makes it a favourable material for the skeleton of the rapidly growing embryo. The cartilaginous skeletal elements present in fetal life are subsequently replaced by bone.

Hyaline cartilage, the most widely distributed form, has a pearl-gray semitranslucent matrix containing randomly oriented collagen fibrils but relatively little elastin. It is normally found on surfaces of joints and in the cartilage making up the fetal skeleton. In elastic cartilage, on

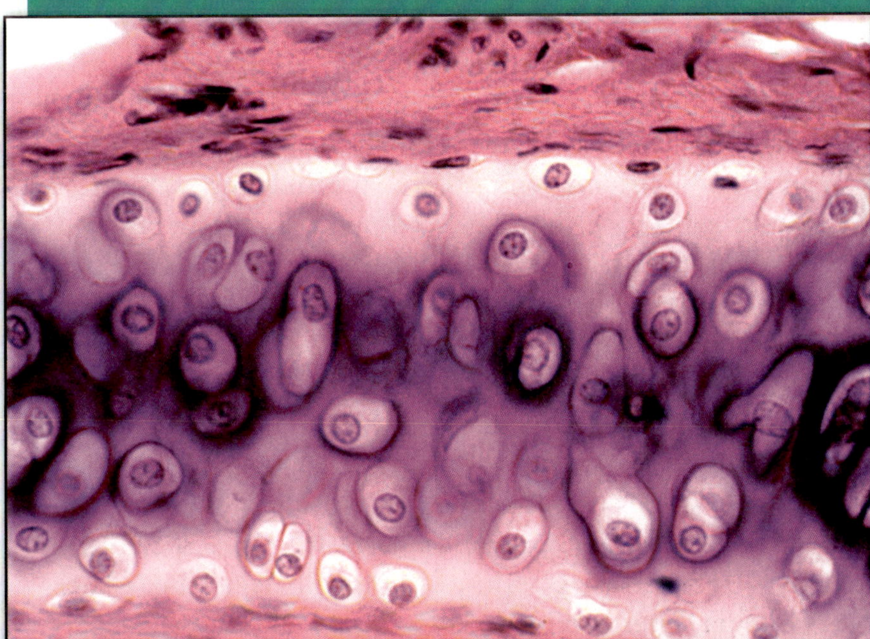

A cross section of hyaline cartilage. Joint surfaces throughout the human body are covered by hyaline cartilage, as are the developing skeletons of human fetuses. Dr. Fred Hossler/Visuals Unlimited/Getty Images

the other hand, the matrix has a pale yellow appearance owing to the abundance of elastic fibres embedded in its substance. This variant of cartilage is more flexible than hyaline cartilage and is found principally in the external ear and in the larynx and epiglottis. The third type, called fibrocartilage, has a large proportion of dense collagen bundles oriented parallel. Its cells occupy lacunae that are often arranged in rows between the coarse bundles of collagen. It is found in intervertebral disks, at sites of attachment of tendons to bone, and in the articular disks of certain joints. Any cartilage type may have foci of calcification.

Ligament

Ligaments are tough fibrous bands of connective tissue that serve to support the internal organs and hold bones together in proper articulation at the joints. A ligament is composed of dense fibrous bundles of collagenous fibres and spindle-shaped cells known as fibrocytes, with little ground substance (a gel-like component of the various connective tissues). Ligaments may be of two major types: white ligament and yellow ligament. White ligament is rich in collagenous fibres, which are sturdy and inelastic. Yellow ligament is rich in elastic fibres, which are quite tough even though they allow elastic movement.

At joints, ligaments form a capsular sac that encloses the articulating bone ends and a lubricating membrane, the synovial membrane. Sometimes the structure includes a bursa—a recess, or pouch, lined by synovial tissue. Other ligaments fasten around or across bone ends in bands, permitting varying degrees of movement, or act as tie pieces between bones (such as the ribs or the bones of the forearm), restricting inappropriate movement.

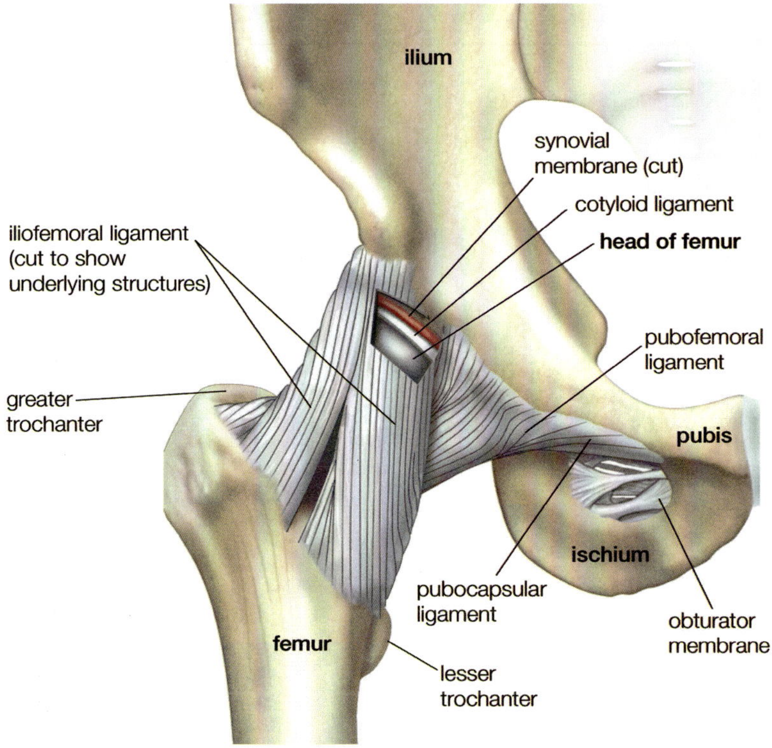

Anterior view of the hip and pelvis, showing attachment of ligaments to the femur, ilium, ischium, and pubis. Encyclopædia Britannica, Inc.

Tendon

Tendons are tissues that attach muscles to other body parts, usually bones. Tendons are the connective tissues that transmit the mechanical force of muscle contraction to the bones. The tendon is firmly connected to muscle fibres at one end and to components of the bone at its other end. Each tendon is composed of dense fibrous connective tissue made up primarily of spindle-shaped fibroblasts and of collagenous fibres. The tendon is attached to the bone by collagenous fibres (Sharpey fibres) that continue into the matrix of the bone. The composition of a tendon is similar to that of ligaments and aponeuroses. The great tensile strength of tendons, which is necessary to withstand the stresses generated by muscular contraction, is made possible by the large quantity of collagenous fibres, which are remarkably tough and strong.

Bone and Periosteum

Like other connective tissues, bone consists of cells, fibres, and ground substance, but, in addition, the extracellular components are impregnated with minute crystals of calcium phosphate in the form of the mineral hydroxyapatite. The mineralization of the matrix is responsible for the hardness of bone. It also provides a large reserve of calcium that can be drawn upon to meet unusual needs for this element elsewhere in the body. The structural organization of bone is adapted to give maximal strength for its weight-bearing function with minimum weight. There are bones strong enough to support the weight of an elephant and others light enough to give internal support and leverage to the wings of birds.

The periosteum forms the dense fibrous membrane covering the surfaces of bones. It consists of an outer fibrous layer and an inner cellular layer (cambium). The outer layer is composed mostly of collagen and contains nerve fibres that cause pain when the tissue is damaged. It also contains many blood vessels, branches of which penetrate the bone to supply the osteocytes, the mature cells of bone tissue. These perpendicular branches pass into the bone along channels known as Volkmann canals to the vessels in the haversian canals, which run the length of the bone. Fibres from the inner layer also penetrate the underlying bone, serving with the blood vessels to bind the periosteum to the bone as Sharpey fibres.

The inner layer of the periosteum contains osteoblasts (bone-producing cells) and is most prominent in fetal life and early childhood, when bone formation is at its peak. In adulthood these cells are less evident, but they retain their functional capacities and are vital to the constant remodeling of bone that goes on throughout life. In the event of bone injury, they proliferate greatly to produce new bone in the repair process. Following an injury such as a fracture, the periosteal vessels bleed around the traumatized area, and a clot forms around the fragments of bone. Within two days the osteoblasts multiply, and the cambium expands to become many cell layers thick. The cells then begin to differentiate and lay down new bone between the ends of the fracture.

The periosteum covers all surfaces of the bone except for those capped with cartilage, as in the joints, and sites for attachment of ligaments and tendons. Fibrous cartilage often takes the place of the periosteum along grooves where tendons exert pressure against the bone. The periosteum on the inner surface of the skull is also modified to some extent as it joins the dura mater, the membrane protecting the brain.

CHAPTER 3

Embryology and Biodynamics of Skin and Connective Tissue

A deeper understanding of the structure and function of human skin and connective tissue can be gained by exploring the embryological development and evolutionary history of these tissues. (Embryology is the study of the formation and development of an embryo and fetus.) Throughout the evolution of land vertebrates and archaic humans, skin changed dramatically with respect to texture, hair covering, pigmentation, and even cellular composition. The properties that characterize the skin layers of modern humans have been influenced in large part by adaptations to environmental conditions.

Human skin and connective tissue are also characterized by a variety of biodynamic properties. For example, skin plays an important role in protection and communication, and connective tissue is vital to movement. Skin is further distinguished by its function as a sense organ—it has the ability to detect touch, pain, and fluctuations in temperature. Pigmentation is also considered to be a biodynamic property of skin.

EMBRYOLOGY AND EVOLUTION

The skin of vertebrates begins to form early in embryonic development, from a superficial germ layer, the ectoderm. The middle germ layer, or mesoderm, proliferates cells rapidly from segmental building blocks, called somites. The somites then migrate in order to lie directly under the outer ectodermal covering. These two embryonic layers—ectoderm and mesoderm—ultimately give rise to the adult skin. The ectoderm produces the epidermis and its derivatives, and the mesoderm produces the dermis.

The human fetus, at least, produces a specialized temporary embryonic skin, known as the periderm. For much of the second trimester of gestation, the periderm consists of cells with projecting globules covered with small protrusions, or microvilli. These cells are subsequently sloughed off as the stratum corneum is formed underneath them.

Differentiation of embryonic tissues proceeds rapidly during the early course of development, and much of what will become adult skin structures—including the glands and appendages—is laid down before the animal is born, often in a latent stage, to resume development later.

As a surface constantly exposed to the environment, the epidermis has undergone more adaptive changes during evolution than any other portion of the skin. Ancestral vertebrates, aquatic and fishlike, were buffeted by water, which kept the living surfaces moist. The movement to land was gradual and fraught with risk. Amphibians were among the first vertebrates to explore the terrestrial environment. Many evolved a semiaquatic lifestyle, exploiting the land for most of their activities but returning to the water for reproduction. Some remained entirely aquatic, and others adapted to a strictly terrestrial life. Their epidermises reflected such habits. Aquatic amphibians developed a thin, slimy, dull skin densely covered with mucous glands. In contrast, terrestrial forms acquired a thicker, horny, heavily pigmented skin dotted with poison glands.

The reptiles became even more independent of the water. Their skins grew tough, horny, and dry

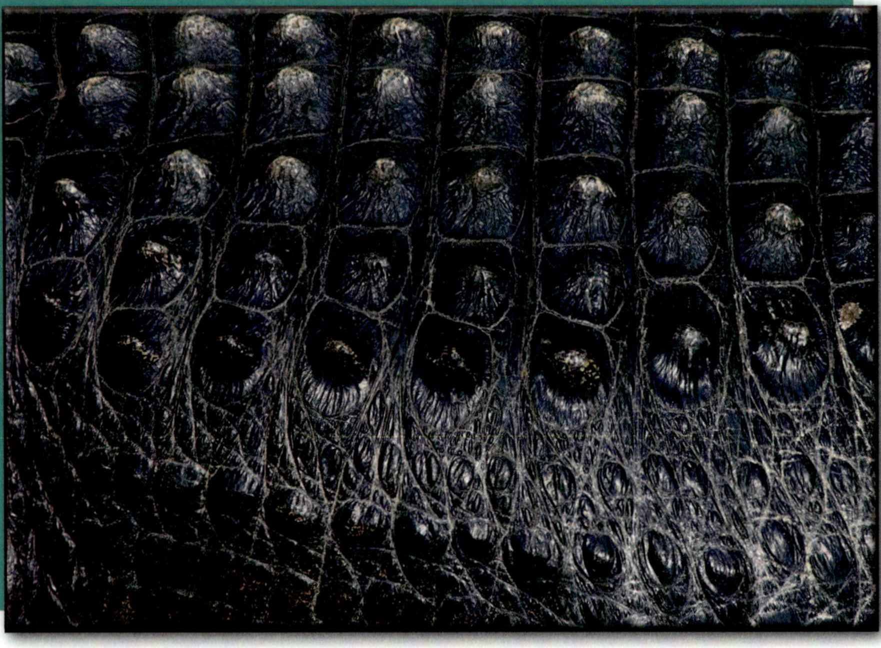

Close-up of alligator skin. The external covering of reptiles is dry and composed of scales made of keratin. It bears few glands or none at all. The epidermis experiences growth cycles, and outer layer cells die and harden into a tough and horny surface. © Corbis

and sometimes received bony contributions from the dermis. Birds evolved a loose, dry skin covered with feathers for insulation and for airfoils and water foils. Finally, mammals adopted a dry, elastic skin, more or less covered with hair. The range of mammalian skin, from smooth (glabrous), as in the cetaceans (whales, dolphins, and porpoises), to densely hairy, as in Arctic bears, is associated with the dispersion of mammals into a wide range of habitats.

Embryological Tissues

The ectoderm is the outermost of the three germ layers, or masses of cells, which appears early in the development of an animal embryo. In vertebrates, ectoderm subsequently gives rise to hair, skin, nails or hooves, and the lens of the eye; the epithelia (surface, or lining, tissues) of sense organs, the nasal cavity, the sinuses, the mouth (including tooth enamel), and the anal canal; and nervous tissue, including the pituitary body and chromaffin tissue (clumps of endocrine cells). In adult cnidarians (e.g., corals, hydras, and jellyfish) and ctenophores (comb jellies), the body-covering tissue, or epidermis, is occasionally called ectoderm.

The outer portion of an embryo, from which the skin and subcutaneous tissues are developed, is known as the dermatome. Postnatally, the dermatome forms the areas of skin supplied by the branches of a single dorsal root ganglion (a dense group of nerve-cell bodies). In the developing embryo the dermatome arises from one of the three segments (somites) of the mesoderm, the middle layer of embryonic tissue.

Dermatomes are arranged with considerable regularity in the vertebrate trunk, although there is some overlap with similar areas above and below. Because each dermatomic area of skin is innervated by branches of nerves originating from a single dorsal root ganglion, the loss of sensation in an area of skin can be traced to a specific spinal nerve, facilitating the diagnosis of spinal cord injuries and certain neurological diseases.

A somite is a longitudinal series of blocklike segments into which the mesoderm, the middle layer of tissue, on either side of the embryonic spine becomes divided. Collectively, the somites constitute the vertebral plate. Out of the somites arise the sclerotome, forerunner of the bodies and neural arches of the vertebrae; the dermatome, precursor of the connective tissue of the skin; and the myotome, or primitive muscle, from which the major muscles of vertebrates are derived. The term *somite* is also used more generally to refer to a body segment, or metamere, of a segmented animal.

The mesoderm, as already mentioned, is the middle of the three germ layers, lying between the ectoderm and endoderm, which appears early in the development of an animal embryo. In vertebrates it subsequently gives rise to muscle, connective tissue, cartilage, bone, notochord, blood, bone marrow, lymphoid tissue, and to the epithelia of blood vessels, lymphatic vessels, body cavities, kidneys, ureters, gonads (sex organs), genital ducts, adrenal cortex, and certain other tissues.

BIODYNAMIC PROPERTIES

The vertebrate skin—despite its variety—serves the two common functions of protection from, and communication with, the environment. In all land vertebrates the uppermost layers of the skin are dead, but the dermis is richly endowed with living tissue that can respond rapidly to change. A variety of nerve endings constantly report current conditions, and the body makes continuous adjustments in response.

It has been said that the skin is the largest and most versatile organ of the animal body. It shields against injury, against foreign matter and disease organisms, and against potentially harmful rays of the Sun. It also regulates internal body temperature through its insulating ability and its influence on blood flow. Further, it embodies the sense of touch and adorns the body. Its contours, colour, patterns, and composition aid in species recognition and sexual attraction.

The effectiveness of the skin as a barrier, however, is not complete. Noxious substances that can gain entry evoke an immune response, and the dermis reddens with the rush of blood to the site. Heat also causes expansion of the dermal blood vessels—and in humans and in horses stimulates the sweat glands to heightened activity—thus increasing the loss of body heat. Conversely, cold causes contraction of the vessels and initiates shivering, thereby conserving heat in the first instance and generating it in the second.

The skin is host to a number of microorganisms, especially bacteria and fungi. It is, however, an unstable environment for this population, which lives on the dead epidermal surface that is periodically sloughed off. A normal microcosm exists on most epidermal surfaces. Over the course of evolution an alliance has been established between the skin biota and the epidermal "host," which tends to stabilize the surface. Thus, anything that disrupts the skin biota encourages an imbalance and a potential flare-up of certain microorganisms over others.

Cutaneous Sense Organs

The skin has both free nerve endings and so-called corpuscular endings, which include nonnervous elements. The corpuscular endings are further differentiated as encapsulated or nonencapsulated receptors.

Free nerve endings occur in the epidermis, in the superficial dermis, where they are arranged in tufts, and in hair follicles. Merkel cells, which are found in the basal layer of the epidermis, are an example of nonencapsulated corpuscular receptors. The most striking example of an encapsulated receptor is the Pacinian corpuscle, an ovoid structure that is about one millimetre in length and lamellated in section, like an onion. These receptors can be found deep in the dermis. Various other dermal sense organs—for example, Golgi-Mazzoni corpuscles, Krause end bulbs, Meissner corpuscles, and Ruffini endings—have also been described.

It can easily be demonstrated that touch, cold, warmth, and pain are each perceived in separate points on the skin surface. The various end organs were at one time, therefore, somewhat arbitrarily assigned as monitors of one or another of these qualities. A difficulty was that many of the receptors are present only in glabrous skin, even though hairy skin in similarly perceptive. These earlier ideas were undoubtedly too simple, but electrophysiologists have confirmed the view that the various end organs respond to specific stimuli. The functional existence of mechanoreceptors, thermoreceptors, and pain receptors has been established, though only some of these can be identified with classical end organs. The Merkel cells and Ruffini endings, for example, are "slowly adapting" mechanoreceptors. The Meissner, Pacinian, and Golgi-Mazzoni corpuscles and the hair follicle receptors are "rapidly adapting" mechanoreceptors.

As already noted, studies of cutaneous sensitivity yield evidence that the human senses number more than five. There is evidence for two pressure senses (for light and for deep stimulation), for two kinds of temperature sensitivity (warm and cold), and for a pain sense. In the 1880s, findings that the human skin is punctate (selectively sensitive at different points) gave clear indication of a dissociation among functions once grouped together as the sense of touch. Mapping the skin with a fine bristle or with a narrow-tipped (warm or cold) cylinder showed that there are different spots of maximum sensitivity to pressure, warm temperatures, and cold temperatures. When stimulated between the spots on the skin, no such sensations were reported. Pain spots also can be located with a finely pointed needle, but the punctate character is less striking since pain seems to be widespread when stimulus intensity is increased. The number of spots is greatest for pain, next for touch, then for cold, and least for warm.

Nerve Function

Microscopic examination of the skin reveals a variety of nerve terminals including free nerve endings (which are most common), Ruffini endings, and encapsulated endings, such as Pacinian corpuscles, Meissner's corpuscles, and Krause end bulbs.

In laboratory animals some nerve endings seem to respond only to one type of stimulus (e.g., to pressure stimuli of very light weight or to slight temperature changes). Others exhibit a broad range of sensitivity. Some receptors show combined sensitivity to both temperature and pressure. In some cases only special types of mechanical stimulation (such as rubbing) may be effective. Furthermore, there is extensive overlap in the areas of skin (receptor fields) for individual nerve fibres, suggesting a neural integration of overlapping afferent inputs of skin nerves.

On the other hand, some tactile receptors (e.g., Pacinian corpuscles) respond only to mechanical deformation. A Pacinian corpuscle is an onion-shaped structure of nonneural (connective) tissue built up around the nerve ending that reduces the mechanical sensitivity of the nerve terminal itself. If the onionlike capsule is entirely removed, mechanical sensitivity not only remains but is somewhat greater than when the capsule is present.

In addition to the differences in the sensory end structures of the skin, the afferent nerve fibres (axons) from them also show diversity. The nerve fibres range in size from large myelinated (sheathed) axons of 10 to 15 micrometres (millionths of a metre) in diameter to extremely small unmyelinated fibres measuring only tenths of micrometres across. Fatter axons tend to conduct nerve impulses more rapidly than do small fibres. When axons of different diameters form a single bundle (a nerve), they constitute a so-called mixed nerve. Thus, electrical records from a mixed nerve show what are labeled A (fast), B (medium), and C (slow) components that reflect the typical speeds at which axons of different diameters conduct. Although such specialized capsules, such as Pacinian corpuscles, tend to be associated with larger diameter axons, and temperature-sensitive endings tend to be associated with medium-size fibres, a unique relation of each of the skin modalities with one of the A, B, or C fibre groups cannot be supported. All of the cutaneous senses seem to be associated with some fibres of all diameters. Furthermore, the C fibres (once thought to be restricted to the pain function) display quite specific sensitivities to nonpainful stimuli applied to the skin.

A major neural pathway for tactile impulses runs along the back (in the dorsal columns) of the spinal cord. Afferent fibres enter the cord from the cutaneous nerves and ascend without synaptic break in one (the ipsilateral) dorsal column. This is a very rapidly conducting pathway shared by fibres that mediate sensations of deep pressure and kinesthesis. Other tactual, temperature, and pain information crosses the spinal cord close to the level of entry of the sensory fibres and ascends to the brain in contralateral pathways of the cord (the lateral and ventral spinothalamic tracts).

Each of the nerves distributed along the spinal cord contains a sensory bundle that serves a well-defined strip of skin (a dermatome) about 2.5 cm (1 inch) wide or more on the body surface. Successive spinal nerves

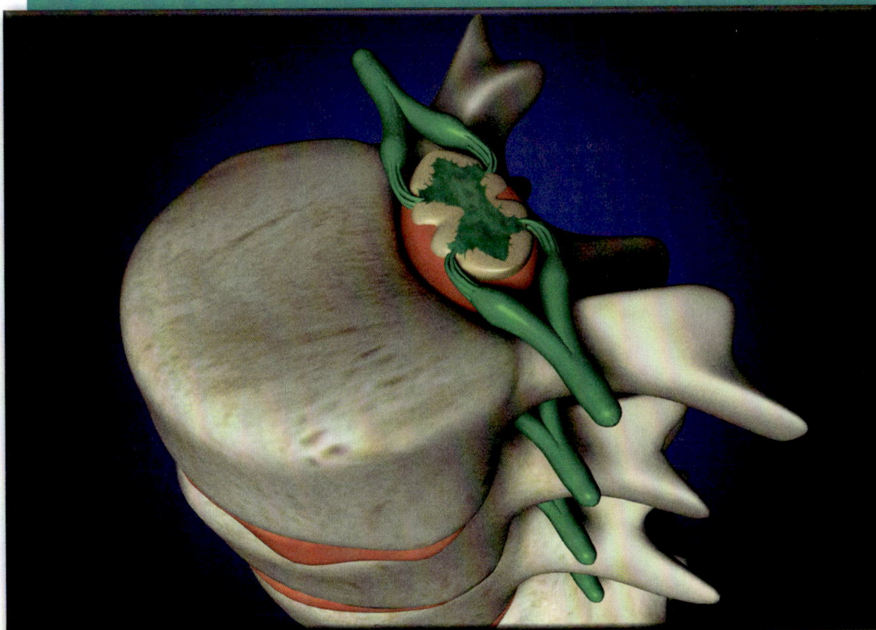

Illustration of a human spinal cord, with nerves highlighted in green. Tactile impulses travel from the skin to the nerves, which relay information through the spinal column to the brain. Shutterstock.com

overlap, so that each place on the skin represents two and sometimes three dermatomes. This yields a segmented pattern of strips over the body from head to toe. All dermatomes feed into a single relay centre (the sensory thalamus) deep within the brain, where there is a precise three-dimensional layout of tactile sensitivity at the body surface. The neurons in this part of the thalamus (the ventral posterolateral nucleus) are specific to particular skin senses (such as pressure) and form small and precise receptor fields. Pathways from the specific ventral posterolateral thalamus end (or project) in a narrow band of the cerebral cortex (the posterior rolandic cortical sensory area) where there is a point-for-point representation of the body surface on the cortical surface. There is a second more diffuse thalamic system (in the posterior thalamic nuclei) where the receptor fields are large, perhaps bilateral, on the left and right sides, perhaps including one whole side of the body. The receptor fields here and the types of stimuli to which they respond are not clearly delineated. The cortical projection of the posterior thalamic system is less well charted than that of the ventral posterolateral thalamus. Thus, there appears to be a dissociation between tactual structures that are highly specific and those that are more generalized.

The dissociation of cutaneous senses is demonstrated in the course of some diseases. For example, in syringomyelia, degeneration of the central canal of the spinal cord leads to loss of pain and temperature sensitivity. Nevertheless, the patient still can experience pressure. In some instances there may be a complete absence of pain sensitivity with disastrous consequences such as bruises, cuts, or even the loss of body parts. Still other instances of dissociation of pain versus pressure occur in surgical procedures (such as tractotomy) in which spinal tracts or parts of the nerves leading into the brainstem are selectively cut. Such operations are designed specifically to relieve pain without unduly diminishing pressure sensitivity.

Tactile Psychophysics

The mixture of sensitivities within a given patch of skin provides a basis for the concept of adequate stimulation. Sometimes, for example, a cold spot responds to a very warm stimulus, and one experiences what is called paradoxical cold. The sensation of heat from a hot stimulus presumably arises from the adequate stimulation of warmth receptors combined with the inadequate or inappropriate (although effective) stimulation of cold and pain receptors.

The ability to detect pressure (i.e., pressure threshold) generally appears when a tension of about 0.85 gram per square mm (equivalent to about 1.2 pounds per square inch) of skin surface is applied on the back of the hand. Thus, a force of 85 mg applied to a stimulus hair (or bristle) of 0.1 square mm is just about enough to elicit the experience of pressure. The energy of impact at pressure threshold is much greater than that required for hearing or seeing, the skin requiring approximately 100,000,000 times more energy than the ear and 10,000,000,000 times more energy than the eye. Differential pressure discrimination (the ability to detect just noticeable differences in intensity) requires changes of roughly 14 percent at maximum sensitivity.

Adaptation to pressure is well known. One's awareness of a steadily applied bristle fades and ultimately disappears. As a result people are rarely aware of the steady pressure of their clothing unless movement brings about a change in stimulation. Most dramatic and perhaps best known among tactile experiences is adaptation to thermal stimulation. Continued presentation of a warm or cold stimulus leads to reduction or disappearance of the initial sensation and an increase in threshold values. Total obliteration of thermal sensation through adaptation occurs in the range from about 16 to 42 °C (61 to 108 °F). If one hand is placed in a bowl of hot (40 °C [104 °F]) water and adapted to that, and at the same time the other hand is adapted to cold (20 °C [68 °F]) water, then when both hands are simultaneously placed in lukewarm (30 °C [86 °F]) water, the previously cooled hand feels warm and the other hand feels cold. Both types of temperature receptors show adaptation. Cold receptors are characterized by an electrical discharge on sudden cooling, normally showing no response to sudden warming. Similar electrical responses are produced by warmth receptors. Both receptors show steady discharges selectively depending on temperature. Maximum discharge typically occurs between 38 and 43 °C (100 and 109 °F) for individual warmth receptors and between 15 and 34 °C (59 and 93 °F) for cold receptors.

Pain is the least understood among all of the human senses. The pattern of stimulation is more crucial in pain than in any other sense. A single brief electric shock to the skin or to an exposed nerve may not elicit the experience of pain, yet it tends to become painful upon repetitive stimulation. Cutaneous pain is often sensed more sharply than is pain associated with deep tissues of the body (e.g., viscera). Certain areas of the body are relatively analgesic (free of pain). For example, one can bite shallowly into the mucous lining of the cheek without discomfort. The organs of the abdominal cavity are usually insensitive to cutting or burning, but traction or stretching of hollow viscera is painful (as when the stomach is distended by gas). Pain also displays sensory adaptation, although the process appears to be more complex than it is for other sensory modalities. Thus, the intensities of headaches, toothaches, and pains from injury often show cyclic fluctuations, possibly from factors such as changes in blood circulation or in degree of inflammation. The visceral pains, those of dental origin, or of diseased tissues can be reduced by analgesic medications, which tend to be less effective on cutaneous pain.

Pain has a strong emotional context. In certain cases, after frontal lobotomies (a type of brain surgery) have been performed, a person may report that he or she still feels the pain of a pin prick or other irritation but that the pain is not as disturbing or as emotionally disruptive as before the lobotomy. Many phenomena indicate the powerful role of the brain and spinal cord in sensing potentially painful sensory input. According to one theory, a gate control system in the spinal cord modulates sensory input from the skin to determine whether the input is perceived as painful. This theoretical formulation also may account for moment-to-moment fluctuations in the intensity of perceived pain despite the absence of any stimulus change. Such brain-mediated factors as emotional tension or past psychological experiences are thought to influence pain perception by acting upon this spinal gate control system.

Nonpainful tactile pattern stimulation is exemplified by vibration. Different frequencies of vibration are readily discriminated, and a tactile communication system employing vibrations on the skin has been devised, particularly for people who cannot see or hear.

Itching

Itching seems to bear the same relation to pain as tickle does to pressure. Itching, which is also known as pruritus, is a stimulation of free nerve endings, usually at the junction of the dermis and epidermis of the skin, that evokes a desire to scratch. It has been suggested that an itch is a subthreshold sensation of pain. However, although both itch and pain sensations share common nerve pathways, they are generally considered distinct sensory types. Itching evokes a range of sensations, from a tickling that is easily relieved to pathologic itching, which generally indicates a dermatologic or systemic disease.

The typical itching experience usually lasts long enough to demand attention and normally leads to a response such as rubbing or scratching the affected area. A number of skin disorders are accompanied by itching, presumably from a fairly low level of irritation in the affected area (which also may be produced in undiseased skin).

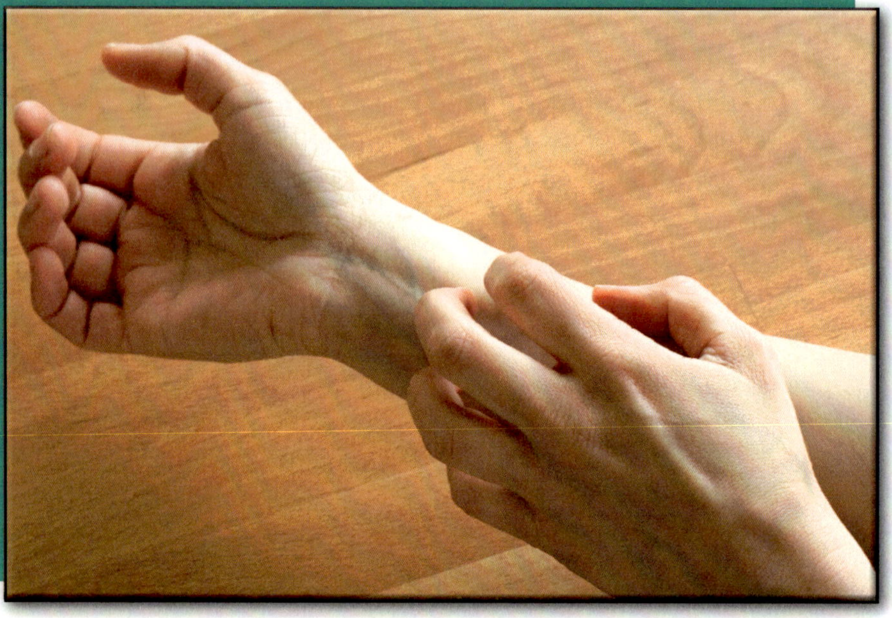

Itching occurs when histamine or some other substance stimulates nerve endings between the dermal and epidermal layers of the skin. Scratching disrupts the impulse, thereby temporarily relieving the itch. © www.istockphoto.com/Heike Kampe

While a single shock by a low-intensity electrical spark normally produces no sensation, a repetitive pattern of such shocks may induce an itch similar to that produced by an insect bite. Itching also may occur as an aftereffect of the sharp pricking sensation produced by single strong shocks, presumably because the nerves continue to produce a patterned afterdischarge following the cessation of the stimulus.

The release of histamine from cells in the epidermis is usually considered to incite most sensations of itching. Scratching may temporarily relieve itching by interrupting the rhythm of nerve impulses or by inflicting transitory damage to the nerves. Persistent scratching produces redness, papules, and crusting of the skin.

Itching associated with skin lesions (such as vesicles and papules) generally indicates a dermatologic disease. Generalized itching without skin lesions can occur in systemic diseases such as those that occur in metabolic and endocrine conditions, malignant cancers, drug reactions, and renal, blood, and liver diseases. Excessive drying of the skin caused by pregnancy, old age, or weather often produces itching. A psychological cause for itching is considered only after all other possibilities have been sufficiently excluded.

No generally accepted therapy exists for the relief of itching, although many have been suggested. Topical anesthetics and other drugs usually have temporary or minor effects. Emollients, applied and blotted dry, may be helpful when applied to wet skin. Antihistamines may also be helpful. At present the choice of therapy usually depends on the underlying cause of the itching, and the focus is primarily on curing the underlying disease rather than the symptom.

Properties of Thermoreceptors

The concept of thermoreceptors derives from studies of human sensory physiology, in particular from the discovery reported in 1882 that thermal sensations are associated with stimulation of localized sensory spots in the skin. Detailed investigations revealed a distinction between warm spots and cold spots—specific places in the human skin that are selectively sensitive to warm or cool stimuli. In general, the specificity of thermoreceptors is quite narrow, in that their nerve endings are excited only, or primarily, by thermal stimuli. However, some thermoreceptors are polymodal, meaning they are capable of responding to both hot and cold stimuli, as well as to certain chemicals, such as capsaicin and menthol, that initiate sensations similar to hot and cold. Some types of cells, including Merkel cells, which are involved in touch reception, and cells on the tongue that are involved in taste, also respond to variations in temperature (although not linearly).

In humans the dynamic relationship between thermoreceptors and other types of sensory receptors is complicated by the concept of conscious sensory specificity, which can differ from biochemical specificity. For example, a thermoreceptor that is excited by cooling and by the application of a chemical (e.g., menthol) might be classified only as a cold thermoreceptor in terms of conscious human sensation. However, biochemically, this receptor plays a role in chemoreception. Conscious sensation is unique in terms of the relationship between thermoreception and mechanoreception. Certain receptor cells in the skin of fishes and amphibians respond both to mechanical and to thermal stimulation. Similar to this, in the skin of cats, monkeys, and humans, certain receptors are excited both by mechanical stimuli and by cooling stimuli. However, these nerve endings are primarily slowly adapting mechanoreceptors that are sensitive to graded pressure on the skin, and their sensitivity to cooling is not linearly related to temperature. In fact, mechanoreceptor nerve fibres that are sensitive to cold have increased spontaneous discharge frequency in the presence of cold stimuli. This is probably responsible for the illusion that a cold metal object (e.g., a silver dollar) placed on the skin seems heavier than the same object at a warm temperature. This phenomenon, known as the silver Thaler illusion, was identified in the 1830s by German anatomist and physiologist Ernst Heinrich Weber. Today, it has been hypothesized that the presence of TRP channels (transient receptor potential channels) in certain mechanoreceptors underlies the phenomenon of spontaneous cold sensitivity. Such molecular evidence has been crucial in improving the understanding of thermoreception and has led to new approaches in the classification of sensory receptors. For example, today receptors sensitive to temperature and other sensory stimuli are more likely to be classified based on genetic similarities and molecular function rather than on the chemical compounds they bind or the stimuli to which they respond.

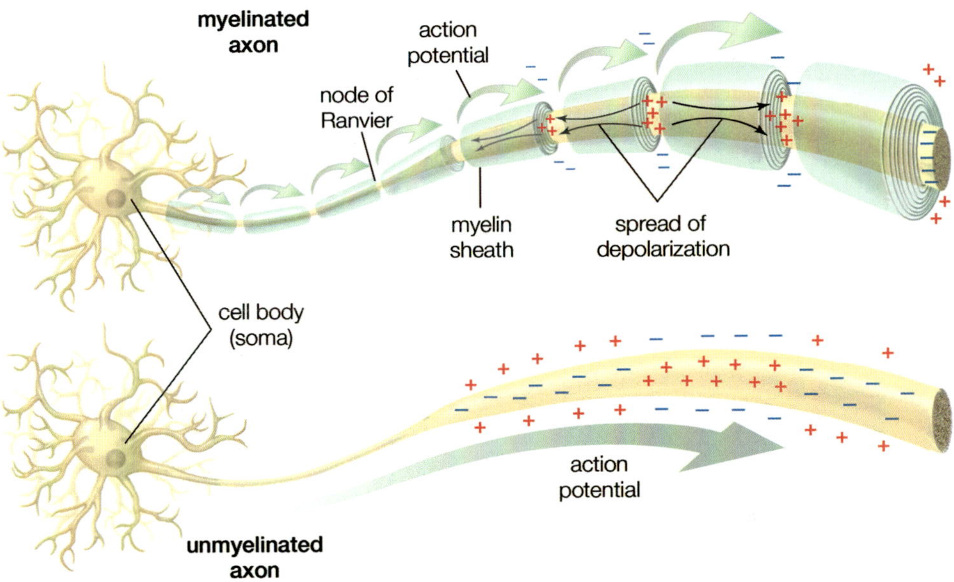

In a myelinated axon, the myelin sheath prevents the local current (small black arrows) from flowing across the membrane. This forces the current to travel down the nerve fibre to the unmyelinated nodes of Ranvier, which have a high concentration of ion channels. Upon stimulation, these ion channels propagate the action potential (large green arrows) to the next node. Thus, the action potential jumps along the fibre as it is regenerated at each node, a process called saltatory conduction. In an unmyelinated axon, the action potential is propagated along the entire membrane, fading as it diffuses back through the membrane to the original depolarized region. Encyclopædia Britannica, Inc.

In general, the properties of thermoreceptors are similar among all species of animals. The electrical signals generated in the peripheral axons of thermoreceptors are brief, all-or-none impulses (action potentials) lasting about one millisecond. The frequency of impulses is affected by environment temperature and by exposure to changes in temperature. For example, at constant temperatures thermoreceptors are continuously active, with the frequency of the steady discharge (static response) depending on the temperature. Thermoreceptors primarily sensitive to cold have increased activity at temperatures cooler than the neutral skin temperature (about 34 °C [93 °F]), and thermoreceptors primarily sensitive to warmth have increased activity at temperatures warmer than neutral skin temperature. The sensitivity of thermoreceptors extends across a continuum of thresholds and response maxima. The static activity of many cold receptors reaches a maximum at temperatures around 20–30 °C (68–86 °F). Some thermoreceptors have lower thresholds (i.e., less than 30 °C [86 °F]) and maximal activity at colder temperatures (i.e., less than 20 °C [68 °F]). For example, a thermoresponsive ion channel known as TRPA1 (subfamily A, member 1) is activated by temperatures below 18 °C (64 °F), which are usually reported as painful. Warm receptors are continuously active at constant temperatures above neutral skin temperature and have response maxima around 41–46 °C (106–115 °F), although, in many cases, warm receptors are inactive at temperatures above 45 °C (113 °F).

Cold receptors respond to sudden cooling with a transient increase in discharge frequency (called the dynamic response) that is directly related to the prior temperature and the magnitude and rate of the temperature decrease. If the cooler temperature is maintained, the discharge frequency adapts to a frequency of static discharge that is directly related to the cooler temperature. When the cold receptor is warmed again, a transient decrease, or inhibition, in discharge frequency occurs, after which the frequency rises again and finally adapts to a new static value. Warm receptors respond in a similar fashion to that of cold receptors, except that they show a dynamic response of increased discharge frequency to warming and a transient inhibition of discharge to cooling. Thus, thermoreceptors are selectively sensitive to specific ranges of temperature, to the rate and direction of temperature change, and to the final temperature. In addition, thermoreceptors are directly sensitive to the absolute temperature at the receptor rather than to the gradient of temperature change within the tissue. There is also evidence that one population of innocuous cool-sensitive thermoreceptors innervates the epidermis, while another population has receptive endings that are situated more deeply in the dermal skin layer.

Pigmentation

The human skin is variously coloured and shows remarkable individual variations even within racial groups. The appearance of the skin is partly due to the reddish pigment in the blood of the superficial vessels. In the main, however, it is determined by melanin, a pigment manufactured by dendritic cells called melanocytes, found among the basal cells of the epidermis. Their numbers in any one region of the body, which range from about 1,000 to more than 2,000 per square millimetre, are roughly the same within and between races. Colour differences are due solely to the amount of melanin produced and the nature of the pigment granules. When the skin becomes tanned on exposure to sunlight, the melanocytes do not increase in number, only in activity.

Melanin

Melanin is a dark biological pigment (biochrome) found in skin, hair, feathers, scales, eyes, and some internal membranes. It is also found in the peritoneum of many animals (e.g., frogs), but its role there is not understood. Melanin is of two kinds: dark brown eumelanin and pale red or yellowish phaeomelanin. Both are formed within the melanocytes by the initial oxidation of the amino acid tyrosine with the aid of the enzyme tyrosinase. After this step, their synthetic pathways diverge. Melanins are conspicuous in dark skin moles of humans, in the black dermal melanocytes (pigment cells) of most dark-skinned peoples, and as brown, diffuse spots in the epidermis.

Melanism refers to the deposition of melanin in the tissues of living animals. The chemistry of the process depends on the metabolism of the amino acid tyrosine, the absence of which results in albinism, or lack of pigmentation. Melanism can also occur pathologically, as in a malignant melanoma, a cancerous tumour composed of melanin-pigmented cells.

Melanic pigmentation is advantageous in many ways: (1) It is a barrier against the effects of the ultraviolet rays of sunlight. On exposure to sunlight, for example, the human epidermis undergoes gradual tanning as a result of an increase in melanin pigment. (2) It is a mechanism for the absorption of heat from sunlight, a function that is especially important for cold-blooded animals. (3) It affords concealment to certain animals that become active in twilight. (4) It limits the incidence of beams of light entering the eye and absorbs scattered light within the eyeball, allowing greater visual acuity. (5) It provides resistance to abrasion because of the molecular structure of the pigment. Many desert-dwelling birds, for example, have black plumage as an adaptation to their abrasive habitat. In addition to protecting the skin from ultraviolet radiation, epidermal pigmentation forms epigamic markings. The heavy pigmentation of the nipples and areolae of breasts, as well as that in the labia minora, penis, and scrotum, is related to sexual communication.

"Industrial" melanism has occurred in certain moth populations, in which the predominant coloration has changed pale gray to dark-coloured individuals. This is a striking example of rapid evolutionary change; it has taken place in less than 100 years. It occurs in moth species that depend for their survival by day on blending into specialized backgrounds, such as lichened tree trunks and boughs. Industrial pollution, in the form of soot, kills lichens and blackens the trees and ground, thus destroying the protective backgrounds of light-coloured moths, which are rapidly picked off and eaten by birds. Melanic moths, by their camouflage, then become selectively favoured. "Industrial" melanic moths have arisen from recurrent mutations and have spread via natural selection.

Melanocytes

Melanocytes are specialized skin cells that produce the pigment melanin. Birds and mammals possess these pigment cells, which are found mainly in the epidermis, though they occur elsewhere—e.g., in the matrix of the hair. Melanocytes are branched, or dendritic, and their dendrites are used to transfer pigment granules to adjacent epidermal cells.

All melanocytes, whether resident in the basal epidermis or in the matrix of the hair, have migrated there during embryonic life from a region known as the neural crest. Each epidermal melanocyte is associated with a group of neighbouring keratinocytes (keratin-synthesizing epidermal cells) into which its dendrites transfer pigment. This structure is known as an epidermal melanocyte unit.

Immunoregulation and Langerhans Cells

Although synthesis of protective keratin is clearly a major function of the epidermis, the discovery of an immunoregulatory role for the epidermis has revolutionized concepts of its importance in the immune defense systems of the host. In addition to melanocytes, human epidermis contains another system of dendritic cells, which do not manufacture pigment. Their distribution extends farther toward the skin surface than that of the pigment cells. After their discovery by the German physician Paul Langerhans in 1868, their function remained obscure until it was realized that they are a vital part of the immunologic mechanism.

Electron microscopic examination has revealed that the morphological hallmark of the Langerhans cell is a unique tennis-racket-shaped organelle, the Birbeck granule. Langerhans cells can be looked upon as "sentinel" cells of the immune system. By virtue of their situation, they are among the first cells to come into contact with foreign particulate substances encountering the skin. Their function is aided by the large surface area created by the dendritic processes of the cell. By means of specialized receptors on the cell membrane, the Langerhans cell recognizes invading as opposed to host molecules. By conveying this information to the lymphoid system, the body is able to mount a defensive immunologic response to the foreign material.

The concept that the role of keratinocytes themselves is confined to the synthesis of a horny protective outer covering for the skin has also become outmoded. Keratinocytes secrete a number of immunostimulatory high-molecular-weight peptides, collectively termed epidermal cytokines. One of these, the epidermal-cell-derived thymocyte-activating factor (ETAF), is also secreted by epidermal Langerhans cells. It has the function of enhancing the immune responsiveness of the lymphoid system as well as apparently being involved in the body's systemic reaction to infection and injury. Because the whole blood volume circulates through the skin every few minutes, immunoregulatory substances released by the cells of the epidermis may have a profound influence on the body's capacity to mount immune responses to viral or bacterial infections or to cancerous growths.

CHAPTER 4

SKIN DISEASES AND INJURIES

A wide variety of diseases or disorders can affect the human skin. Although most diseases involving the skin originate in any of its three layers, such abnormalities are also important factors in the diagnosis of a variety of internal diseases. Thus, there is some truth in the belief that the skin mirrors a person's internal health. Often, the visibility and accessibility of skin make it the first organ of the body to show detectable signs of underlying disease. Skin, however, because of the nature of its exposure to the

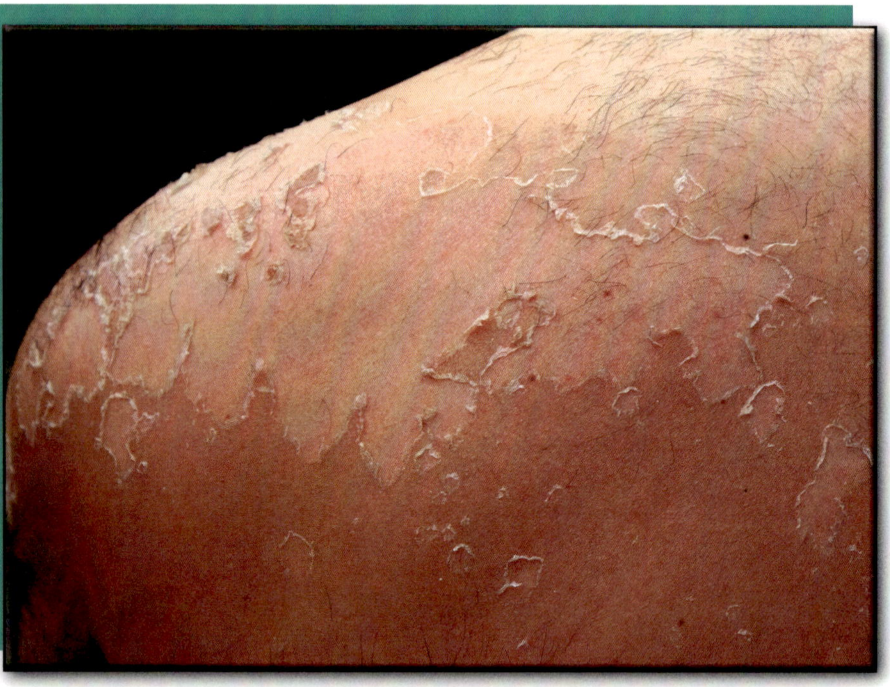

Skin peels from the back of a sunburn victim. The skin has remarkable healing properties and is capable of healing itself quickly after trauma or injury. Shutterstock.com

environment, is highly susceptible to injury, and skin injuries such as minor wounds and bruises are among the most common afflictions of the tissue.

GENERAL FEATURES OF SKIN DISEASE

Like other tissues, skin is afflicted by all types of pathological changes, including hereditary, inflammatory, benign and malignant (neoplastic), endocrine, hormonal, traumatic, and degenerative processes. Thus, abnormalities of the skin frequently suggest metabolic, malignant, and glandular diseases. Emotions affect the health of the skin as well.

The reaction of the skin to diseases and disorders differs from that of other tissues in many ways. For example, extensive inflammation of the skin may affect metabolism within other organs and systems of the body, causing anemia, circulatory collapse, disorders of body temperature, and disturbance of water and electrolyte balance in the blood. The skin has such vigorous healing properties, however, that widespread injury, as in thermal burns, may be followed by a marked degree of regrowth of the injured or diseased areas, with a disproportionally small degree of scarring.

The skin has an inherent region-specific anatomical diversity that may profoundly modify the appearance of a rash. This is apparent when skin transplanted from one area of the body to another (other than a symmetrically opposite area) retains the morphological characteristics of the donor area. Thus, the morphology of eczema or of the inflammatory condition lichen planus on the palms and soles may bear little or no resemblance to the same disease in the same individual on the face or scalp. In these instances a biopsy shows the abnormalities of the cells of the skin and the pattern and distribution of any invading cells. The ability to identify immunoreactants (immunoglobulins, or antibodies, that react with specific invading agents, or antigens) in skin biopsies has greatly increased the accuracy of the diagnosis of inflammatory disorders and has clarified their immunologic basis, especially in the blistering disorders.

The classification of hereditary skin disorders generally has been based upon gross morphological, histological, and electron microscopic findings. However, because a skin disease may not always have a characteristic presentation, the specific diagnosis sometimes has been in doubt. Better understanding of the biochemical defects underlying hereditary skin disorders now allows these conditions to be diagnosed with more precision. One subset of the ichthyoses, a group of sometimes disabling genetic skin disorders, may thus be delineated from other members of the group, based on biochemical detection of a specific enzyme defect (reduced steroid sulfatase enzyme).

Skin diseases in which there is an overproduction of epidermal cells or a disorganization of their differentiation often show scaling. Simple benign hyperplasia (overgrowth) of the epidermis such as is commonly seen in infantile eczema often appears as lichenification, a term used to describe a thickening of the epidermis in which the normal surface markings of the skin are greatly exaggerated. Chronic benign or malignant proliferative dermatoses involving the epidermis often have a rough warty surface caused by overproduction by the epidermal cells of keratin.

There are relatively few skin diseases in which inflammation, including responses to physical injury (such as sunburn), allergy, and infections (such as boils and cold sores), does not play a part. Even cancerous lesions of the skin frequently show some degree of inflammatory response. Inflammation is usually the result of the release of chemical mediators in the skin. These mediators include histamine, which is stored in a preformed state in the skin, and peptides (kinins) and fatty acids (prostaglandins and leukotrienes), which are formed enzymatically in response to injury. In some skin diseases inflammation is the major factor in the morphological appearance of the rash (for example, acute allergic contact dermatitis).

The most important features of inflammation include redness, caused by dilation of blood vessels; heat, caused by increased blood flow; swelling, caused by leakage of fluid from the small blood vessels; and pain or itching. In addition, the affected skin may feel indurated (hardened) because of the deposition of the coagulation protein fibrin and the infiltration by inflammatory blood cells (lymphocytes, histiocytes, and polymorphonuclear leukocytes). Medications designed to counteract inflammation in the skin may antagonize the effects of mediators (e.g., antihistamines). Nonsteroidal anti-inflammatory drugs of the type effective in arthritis, including aspirin and indomethacin, have proved to be of little or no value in the treatment of inflammatory skin diseases.

Whealing reactions (hives, nettle rash, urticaria) constitute a special form of inflammation in which vascular changes predominate, with little or no inflammatory cellular reaction. Localized fluid accumulation (edema) causes the development of a short-lived wheal associated with intense itching. Its appearance frequently indicates an underlying allergic cause. Intense inflammation may occasionally lead to the formation of blisters, caused by the effects of enzymes released from inflammatory cells, from the resident cells of the skin, or from blood plasma components. These enzymes cause the breakdown of proteins responsible for the structural integrity of the skin. In some blistering (bullous) skin diseases (such as pemphigus), the development of large blisters is the predominant morphological feature.

Inflammatory diseases of the dermis often evoke a secondary proliferative and scaly response in the epidermis. Dermal inflammatory disorders may be acute, as in hemolytic (blood-cell destroying) streptococcal infections leading to cellulitis (diffuse inflammation of the connective tissues), or chronic and granulomatous, as in chronic cutaneous tuberculosis (lupus vulgaris). In the first instance the changes of acute inflammation are present but there is normally no epidermal change. In the second, the skin is hardened and thickened, and it has a brownish appearance under the microscope.

The intrinsic colour of normal skin is pale yellow, but this colour is modified by pigments—both by melanin and by hemoglobin. The intensity of the brown hue conferred by melanin depends on the distribution of the melanin granules within the cells. All races have the same number of melanocytes, although melanin is produced and distributed through the epidermis more efficiently in blacks. Increased melanin pigmentation is a common reaction to prolonged inflammation of the skin. The intensity and shade of pink depend on the state of the cutaneous circulation. When blood vessels are dilated with increased blood flow, as in an inflammatory disorder, the skin is bright red. The vasodilation associated with stagnant blood flow, as in excessive cooling of the skin, gives the skin a purplish hue.

The predominant symptom of skin disease is itching. Although an itching sensation may result in healthy skin from a direct conversion of very light pressure (light stroking of the skin of the lips is a good example), in most skin diseases itching is caused by the release of pharmacological mediators, such as histamine. When itching occurs in normal-appearing skin, as is the case in liver or kidney disease, the itching is probably due to an abnormal accumulation of metabolic products in the skin.

ERYTHEMA

Erythema is any abnormal redness of the skin. It is caused by dilation and irritation of the superficial capillaries. The augmented flow of blood through them imparts a reddish hue to the skin. Erythema may arise from a great variety of causes and disease conditions. Blushing is a transient form of erythema.

From a medical point of view, the two major erythemas are erythema multiforme and erythema nodosum. Erythema multiforme is characterized by the sudden eruption of crops of red or violet flat spots, wheals, papules (small solid elevations), and vesicles (blisters), the characteristic lesions often having a concentric, or target, pattern. The skin on the palm of the hand and the mucous surfaces, especially the mouth and eyelids, are commonly involved. Erythema multiforme is believed to be a symptom complex that is secondary to a wide variety of underlying disease states. It may run a severe course and become life-threatening; in mild cases, the eruption is prone to recur. Variable success in treatment is obtained with the use of corticosteroid hormones.

Erythema nodosum is a hypersensitivity reaction most commonly associated with streptococcal infection, drugs (particularly oral contraceptives), and sarcoidosis (a systemic disease characterized by the formation of granulation, or scarlike, tissue). It is marked by the sudden onset of multiple, red, painful nodules in the deeper layer of the skin on the external surface of the lower legs. It most often affects young women. The nodules usually disappear spontaneously over a period of several weeks. Recurrences are uncommon. Treatment is usually of the underlying cause and may include complete bedrest, oral salicylates, and—in treatment of sarcoidosis—systemic corticosteroids.

Those erythematous conditions that are directly caused by specific agents include endemic erythema, or pellagra, due to a dietary deficiency of the vitamin niacin; and erythema ab igne, due to nonburning exposure to radiant heat.

SKIN INJURIES

Common skin injuries include minor open wounds, in which a small break occurs in the skin and, in many cases, in nearby blood vessels, resulting in some amount of bleeding. In contrast, bruises, which are also common injuries and involve the rupture of blood vessels, are considered closed wounds, because the skin layers are left intact. More severe injuries occur in the form of major wounds (such as when a bullet strikes the body), burns, and frostbite. Burns in particular, if serious, may necessitate skin grafting, in which healthy skin is transplanted onto the injured area to aid the healing process.

Skin Wounds and Scars

A wound is a break in the continuity of any bodily tissue due to violence, where violence is understood to encompass any action of external agency, including, for example, surgery. Within this general definition many subdivisions are possible, taking into account and grouping together the various forms of violence or of tissue damage.

The most important distinction is between open and closed wounds. Open wounds are those in which the protective body surface (the skin or mucous membranes) has been broken, permitting the entry of foreign material into the tissues. In closed wounds, by contrast, the damaged tissues are not exposed to the exterior, and the process of repair can take place without the interference that contamination always brings, in greater or lesser degree.

Further divisions may be made on the basis of the mode of production of the wound.

When the skin (or, in the case of injuries of the base of the skull or the sinuses, the mucous membrane) is broken, a wound is exposed to additional hazards, since the tissues may be invaded by foreign material such as bacteria, dirt, and fragments of clothing, which may give rise to serious local or general complications from infection. Furthermore, if the break in the skin is large, the resulting exposure of the wounded tissues to the drying and cooling effects of the air may increase the damage caused by the wounding agent itself.

A needle, a sharp knife, or a rifle bullet that passes through the tissues with ease, dividing them cleanly or separating them, will produce relatively little damage except to those tissues directly in its course. Indeed, unless an important structure is injured, the wounds caused are seldom serious. On the other hand, a bomb fragment, irregular and jagged, will, as it churns and rips through the soft tissues, produce extensive damage for a considerable distance in all directions. Likewise, the injury caused by crushing is frequently serious.

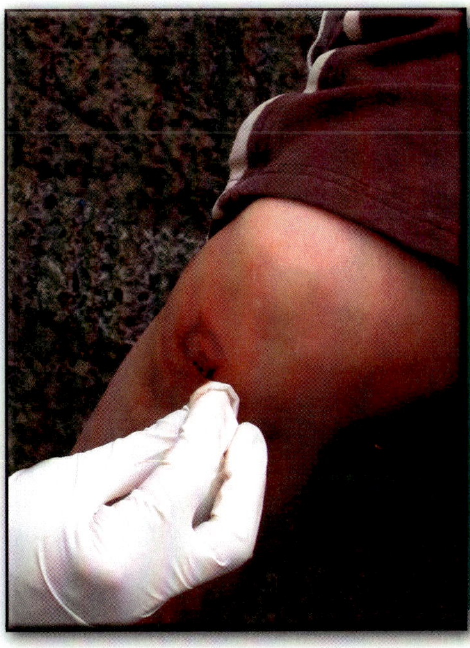

Attending to a scraped, or "skinned," knee. Cuts and scrapes provide an opening for bacteria, and therefore should be thoroughly cleaned to avoid infection. Shutterstock.com

Skin, being sturdy and elastic and well supplied with blood, tolerates injury well and recovers quickly. The subcutaneous fatty tissues are more delicate and more easily deprived of their blood supply. Muscle, likewise, is sensitive to the damaging effect of missiles, being readily torn and unable to survive diminished blood supply for any appreciable time. Muscle, when damaged, is particularly prone to infection.

An injury to bone in an open wound is always serious, for any broken fragment detached from its blood supply will not survive if infection occurs, and it will remain as a foreign body in the wound to cause further complications. Even if the bone is cleanly broken and there are no loose fragments, infection may enter the raw surfaces of the fracture with disastrous results. Clearly the seriousness of a wound is greatly increased if there is injury to a joint, a nerve, a major blood vessel, or an internal organ.

Contamination of a wound may occur at the moment of wounding or at any time thereafter until healing is complete. The effects of various nonbacterial contaminants vary considerably (e.g., organic substances tend to be more irritating than others). In general, the critical factor for nonbacterial contaminants is the extent of the contamination. In the case of bacterial contaminants the type of contaminant is of greater importance. Infection caused by virulent bacteria nourished by dead tissue and organic foreign material in the wound may take several forms, of which the three most important are gas gangrene, the most dreaded, arising almost exclusively in damaged muscle tissue and spreading with alarming rapidity to cause death if unchecked by surgical or medical treatment; infections caused by such organisms as *Streptococcus* and *Staphylococcus* and the coliform bacteria, in which the local production of pus is a prominent feature accompanying a general reaction that may be severe; and tetanus, a treacherous, often fatal infection that becomes evident some days after the wound has occurred, frequently without any marked local manifestations but characterized by generalized muscle spasms.

The final healing of a wound is the result of a series of complex biological events taking place over a long period. Viewed in the simplest way, in an untreated but uncomplicated wound, as from a clean knife cut, the process is as follows: When tissues are cut, the edges of the wound separate, apparently pulled apart by the elasticity of the skin. Blood from the severed blood vessel fills the cavity of the wound and overflows its edges. The blood clots and eventually the surface of the clot dries out and becomes hard, forming a scab. During the first 24 hours the scab shrinks, drawing the edges of the wound closer together. If the scab sloughs off or is removed after about a week, a layer of reddish granulation tissue will be seen to have covered the cut edges of the subcutaneous tissue. Gradually a pearly, grayish, thin membrane extends out from the skin edge, and eventually it covers the whole surface. The actual area of the wound, meanwhile, is steadily reduced by a process of contraction, until finally there is no raw surface to be seen.

The thin linear scar that forms is at first red and raised above the level of the surrounding skin but gradually fades until it is considerably paler than the surrounding skin. For many weeks after the scar forms, this process of contracture continues as is shown by the gradual shortening of the wound. Wounds that cross normal "skin lines" tend, after several months, to widen and become depressed below the level of the surrounding skin. Scars do not tan in sunlight, and they produce neither hair nor sweat, all evidences of the failure of the skin to return to full function.

Microscopically one can observe in the clot the whole process of the development of fibrin that causes the clot to contract, the arrival of the white blood cells and the macrophages that digest the debris in the wound, and the growth of blood capillaries followed by the growth inward of fibrous tissue migrating from the cells on the margin of the wound. The fibres arising from these cells can be identified and seen to increase, eventually filling the wound cavity with a network of interlacing threads of the protein collagen that, influenced by lines of tension, finally range themselves in firm bands. Meanwhile, the surface of the wound is being covered by a process of enlargement and flattening and by multiplication of the preexisting skin cells at the edge of the wound. These covering, or epithelial, cells start very early to spread down into the wound, clearing a way for themselves beneath the scab, perhaps by the production of an enzyme that dissolves the deeper layers of the crust. Eventually the proliferating epithelial sheets from the two sides of the wound coalesce to heal the wound superficially.

In some instances, a scar may become permanent, leaving a mark left on the skin after the healing of a cut, burn, or other area of wounded tissue. As part of the healing process, fibroblasts in adjacent areas of skin produce a fibrous connective tissue made up of collagen. The bundles formed by these whitish, rather inelastic fibres make up the bulk of the scar tissue. Though scar tissues possess networks of small capillaries and are thus supplied with blood, they lack the oil glands and elastic tissue that normally protect the skin against irritation. Consequently, they are often slightly painful or itchy.

Sometimes a scar becomes an excessively thick and fibrous, tumourlike growth called a keloid, which extends beyond the wound's original limits. Another, less serious form of overscarring is that of hypertrophic scars, in which the scar grows overly thick but remains confined within the limits of the wound. Keloids and hypertrophic scars

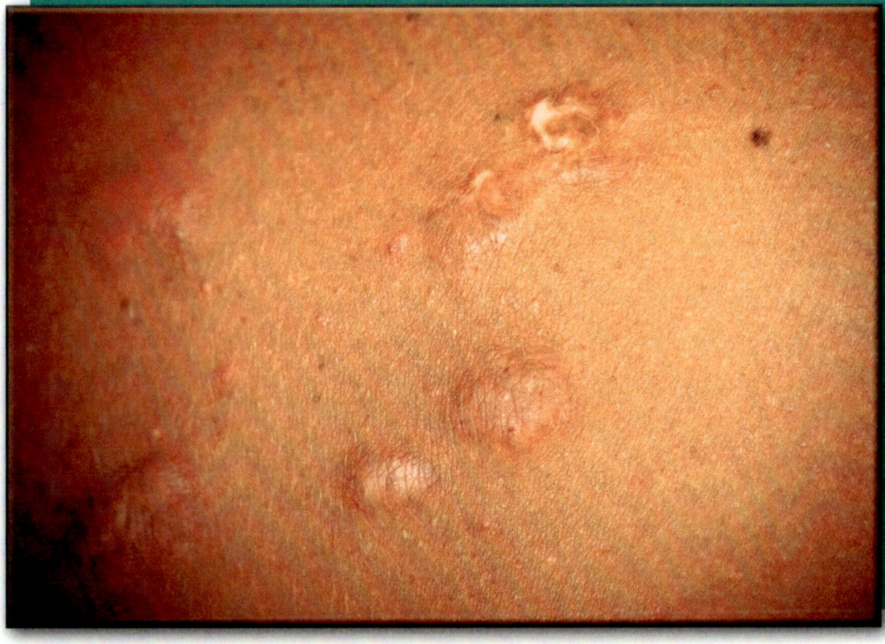

Keloids form when scar tissue thickens and extends beyond a wound site. Surgery, burns, and relatively minor injury caused by procedures such as tattooing and piercing can produce keloids. © www.istockphoto.com/piccerella

are most troublesome when they result from serious burns and cover large areas of the skin. These may inhibit a person's movement, especially around a joint. All scars, but especially those resulting from unaided healing of third-degree burns, also are prone to malignant change.

The treatment of serious or prominent scars is considered by plastic surgeons to be among their most important problems. Dermabrasion (abrading the skin in a controlled manner) can be used to remove unsightly scars that have resulted from surgery or acne. Small scars can best be prevented by keeping a scab from forming on a wound through the use of nonstick bandages. The scars left in the wake of scabs form indentations in the skin.

Bruises

A bruise is a visible bluish or purplish mark or patch occurring beneath the surface of unbroken skin, resulting from the rupture of blood vessels in the deeper layers of subcutaneous tissues. Bruises are usually caused by a blow or pressure but, in aged persons, may occur spontaneously. In healing, the colour of the bruise gradually fades away into a yellowish hue, as a result of the formation of bile pigments and the disintegration and gradual absorption of blood. In hemophilia, a hereditary bleeding disorder, if untreated, bruises of the skin and soft tissue may be almost always present.

Blisters

A blister is a rounded elevation of the skin that contains clear fluid and is caused by a separation either between layers of the epidermis or between the epidermis and the dermis. Blisters are classified as vesicles if they are 0.5 cm (0.2 inch) or less in diameter and as bullae if they are larger. Blisters can commonly result from pressure and friction on sites such as the palms or soles. They are produced when friction causes an upper skin layer to move back and forth over an underlying skin layer. A small gap opens up between them and becomes filled with fluid. Blisters may also occur as symptoms of contact dermatitis, viral infection, or an autoimmune disease, in which case they can appear anywhere on the body.

Blistering usually takes place within the uppermost layer of the skin (epidermis), producing fragile, easily broken blisters. Subepidermal blisters are tenser and are more difficult to break. In either case, the blister fluid is usually clear and colourless. Yellowish fluid is a sign that it contains pus and red that it contains blood. Friction blisters generally heal spontaneously, sometimes leaving a thickened callus; disease blisters may leave scars, particularly when they are located deep in the epidermis.

Calluses and Corns

A callus (also spelled callous) is a small area of thickened skin. Calluses are formed by continued friction, pressure, or other physical or chemical irritants. In response to mild but repeated injury, the cells of the epidermis, the outermost horny layer of the skin, become more active, giving rise to a localized increase in horny tissue on the surface of the skin. Calluses are most frequently seen on the hands and feet. They are usually yellowish white, flat, and painless. When a callus is conical in shape, penetrating into the deeper layer of the skin and causing pain when pressed, it is called a corn.

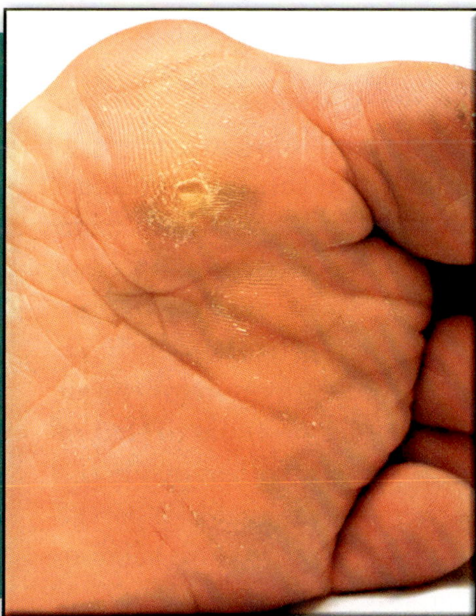

The pressure of walking puts skin of the feet and toes at risk of developing corns, which are calluses with an inner pointed end that presses on sensory nerves, causing pain. Shutterstock.com

Corns can occur in the skin on the foot or toes. They are produced by repeated friction or pressure. Extensive proliferation of the stratum corneum, the horny layer of the epidermis, results in a conical callus with its broad end on the surface and its point directed inward. The dense centre of this cone presses on sensory nerves, causing pain when direct pressure is applied. The corn's surface is usually hard and shiny, but corns between the toes may be soft and soggy from perspiration.

Corns are treated by applying plasters of salicylic or dichloroacetic acid to the site after the core has been removed and the callus pared. They are likely to recur, however, unless the source of friction or pressure is eliminated by a change in footwear or in walking habits. Long-lasting corns may produce a bony spur that must be removed surgically.

Skin Squeeze

Skin squeeze, or body squeeze, is caused by exposure to a pressure less than that of the surrounding environmental pressure. Skin squeeze is most prevalent among pilots and underwater divers working in pressurized suits. In both professions the participants encounter unusual pressures.

In deep-sea diving, especially when the diver is using a pressurized suit and metal helmet supplied with air from the surface, the hazard of body squeeze is common. As a diver goes to underwater depths, the external pressure upon the body increases in proportion to the depth. To prevent injury to the skin and body, the pressure of the air pumped into the suit must at all times be equal to that of the surrounding water. If the air pressure is less inside the suit than the water pressure, the effect is that of a partial vacuum that pulls the body's tissues outward. This vacuum effect causes rupturing of the skin's blood vessels. Pain, tenderness, redness, and swelling of the tissue result. If the vacuum is sufficiently great, the body of the diver may be crushed and sucked up into the helmet. Most cases of skin squeeze occur when there is a blockage in the air hose or malfunction of the air valve so that the pressures cannot be equalized. A diver who falls while under water, so that he or she descends rapidly before the air pressure in the suit can be adjusted, also is subject to body squeeze.

Pilots using pressurized suits can encounter the same difficulties as divers. As one goes higher into space, the external pressure decreases. Upon return to land, the pressure gradually increases once again. If a pressurized suit malfunctions at high altitudes, the pilot can encounter skin squeeze upon descent toward the Earth.

Frostbite

Frostbite is the freezing of living tissue. It occurs whenever heat loss from a tissue is sufficient to permit ice formation. The freezing-thawing process causes mechanical damage to cells (from ice), tissue dehydration, and local oxygen depletion. If not relieved, these conditions lead to disruption of the blood corpuscles, thrombosis (clotting) within the small blood vessels, and tissue gangrene.

Conditions Conducive to Frostbite

Frostbite can occur whenever the ambient temperature falls below 0 °C (32 °F). Without adequate food, clothing, or shelter, heat is lost successively from the interior of the body to the skin, to the layer of still, insulating air surrounding the skin, and finally to the ambient cold air. High-velocity wind blowing away the insulating air cover, as well as the wetting of the skin, hastens the outward transfer of heat. Thus, ice fishermen, hunters, campers, mountaineers, and others exposed to wind and low temperatures may become victims of frostbite.

All too impressive is the injury and death toll from cold during time of war. Armies that suffered as much from the cold as from the enemy include Xenophon's Greeks in Armenia (400 BCE), the Swedish troops of Charles XII in Ukraine (1708), and the army of George

Washington at Valley Forge in America (1777–78). Most classic is the saga of the Napoleonic forces fleeing Russia (1812–13). Pursued by a relentless enemy in the dead of winter, driven onward without food, water, rest, adequate clothing or footwear, many thousands of troops suffered frostbite or froze to death.

Three types of individual physical and health factors can contribute to frostbite. They are (1) conditions encouraging heat loss, (2) mechanical or physical impedance of circulation to the extremities, and (3) problems that decrease the ability of a person to cope with the cold.

Conditions encouraging heat loss are (1) the excessive intake of alcohol, causing capillary dilation, flushing, and dissipation of heat, (2) wet clothing, permitting outward heat conduction, (3) exposed flesh, (4) fever, with radiation of heat, (5) injury, with hemorrhage, anoxia, and shock, causing general body cooling, and (6) overexercise, as in forced survival marches, draining unreplaced calories and heat.

Factors that mechanically impede circulation to the extremities and thus favour cooling and subsequent freezing include (1) tight boots, gloves, or clothing, (2) blood vessel diseases or injuries that diminish the flow of blood to the extremities, causing local tissue oxygen depletion, and (3) constriction of small blood vessels as a result of drug action.

Conditions that decrease the ability of a person to avoid cold insult include (1) emaciation or fatigue, (2) dehydration, a major problem in the cold, with subsequent blood acidity, mental derangement, coma, and death, (3) neuromuscular disease, or previous freezing or nonfreezing cold injury, with resultant sensory loss, predisposing to further cold injury, and (4) psychosis from any cause, allowing behaviour contributory to freezing, with mental disorganization, loss of thermoregulation, and resultant fall of body temperature.

Recognition and Treatment

Frostbite usually affects the toes, fingers, ears, and the tip of the nose first. Before thawing, the affected part is hard, cold, white, or bloodless. The skin is rigid and the depth of freezing difficult to determine. Frostbite is rendered more dangerous by the fact that there is no sensation of pain, and the victim may not even know that he has been frostbitten.

In dealing with frostbite, body temperature is usually restored to as near normal as possible before thawing. Under no circumstances should attempts be made to warm the affected area by rubbing or chafing it, since this can damage the cell structure of the frozen tissues. The old theory that a frostbitten area should be rubbed with snow or ice is similarly false and potentially harmful. Rapid thawing of the hands or feet in warm water baths is a presently favoured method of therapy. Thawing time is determined by the temperature of the bath and the depth of the freezing. Thawing is complete when the tip of the extremity flushes pink or red. (If the affected area remains white after thawing, this means that the cold has so affected local blood vessels that normal circulation has not yet resumed.) After rapid thawing small blisters appear rapidly, spontaneously rupturing in 4 to 10 days. A castlike scab, often black, forms after the blisters rupture. Normal tissue may have already formed below. The thawed part is usually protected to avoid both refreezing and excessive heat. Neither bandages nor dressings are used, and the area is cleansed with benign soaps. Constant digital exercises are performed to preserve joint motion. Early surgical removal of unhealthy tissue (debridement) and amputation is avoided. Whirlpool action will debride devitalized tissues.

Antibiotics are used if necessary. Toxoid booster injections are a recommended precaution. After thawing, further treatment is aimed at the prevention of infection and preservation of function. The outlook is best when the frozen state is of short duration, when the thawing is by rapid rewarming, and when blisters develop early, pink and large, and extend to the tips of the hands or toes. The outlook is uncertain when thawing is spontaneous, as at room temperature, when the frozen state is of long duration, and when the freezing is superimposed on top of a fracture or dislocation. The outlook is poor when thawing is delayed, as in ice and snow, when thawing is by excessive heat (i.e., greater than 46 °C [115 °F]), when the blisters are dark or hemorrhagic and do not extend to the distal tips, when a nonfreezing cold injury is followed by freezing, and when freezing, then thawing by any means, is followed by refreezing. The last two conditions are disastrous and almost always require amputation of the affected part.

Major complications after freezing, and following treatment, may be infection and tissue death, requiring amputation. Less tragic aftereffects are increased sweating, sensory loss, diminished subcutaneous fat pad of the toes and fingers, persistent deep pain, limitation of joint motion, and nail-bed changes. Other permanent effects include fixed scars, wasting of the small muscle, joint deformity, arthritic changes in bone, and neurovascular involvement in the extremities resulting in the inability to protect against lowered temperatures, coupled with increased sensitivity to cold.

Frostbite Prevention

To prevent frostbite, clothing in cold weather should be dry, layered, and with warm, loose hand wear and footwear. Tight, restricting bands should not be worn. Exposed flesh should be protected from the wind: face masks, hoods, and earmuffs are helpful. In cold, an individual must remain alert, avoiding the excessive use of alcohol and drugs inhibiting mental or physical capability.

Should freezing follow an accident, major efforts must be made to avoid further heat loss in order to prevent death. In any situation in which freezing has occurred, thawing should be prevented if refreezing may take place.

Skin Graft

A skin graft is the transplantation of healthy skin from one area of the body to cover and heal a large wound or burn in another area of a similar skin type. The two most widely used techniques are (1) split-thickness grafts, which remove the upper layer (epidermis) and part of the middle layer (dermis) of the skin, allowing the donor site to heal naturally, and (2) full-thickness grafts, which transfer the entire dermis so that the donor site must be surgically closed. An earlier technique, pinch grafting, which used many small grafts instead of one large one, has been abandoned for the most part because of unsightly scarring at the donor site. The most common sites employed as sources for skin grafts are the inner thigh, leg, upper arm, and forearm.

CHAPTER 5

SKIN INFECTIONS AND INFESTATIONS

Healthy skin harbours a resident, harmless bacterial population. However, pathogenic (disease-causing) strains of bacteria such as staphylococci, as well as a host of other agents, including viruses, fungi, and parasites, may inhabit the skin, producing various signs and symptoms of infection or infestation. Some pathogenic bacteria are resistant to antibiotics, the drugs used to treat bacterial infection. Hence, these organisms and the people who carry them pose a serious health hazard, particularly to those with diminished resistance to infection, such as newborn infants and elderly persons. Most infections by resistant organisms occur nosocomially, or in hospitals. Although local measures, such as cleansing of the involved skin, are often effective for minor skin infections, serious infections may require treatment with multiple types of antibiotics. Infections with viruses, fungi, or other agents require different treatment strategies, such as the administration of antiviral or antimicrobial drugs, depending on the type of agent involved.

SIGNS OF INFECTION

Signs of bacterial infection appear after the organisms have been introduced into the dermis. Some organisms, such as staphylococci and streptococci, produce a pustular infection (impetigo, boils) in which the main features are acute inflammation and the accumulation of large numbers of white blood cells as pus. Other organisms, including *Mycobacterium tuberculosis* and *Treponema pallidum* (the spirochete that causes syphilis), may cause more chronic inflammatory changes without pus but involving a characteristic arrangement of mononuclear inflammatory cells called histiocytes. The term *granulomatous* is used to describe this kind of cutaneous reaction to infection. Leprosy is a cutaneous bacterial granulomatous disease in which the causative organism, *Mycobacterium leprae*, resides in the neural tissue in the skin, producing the characteristic features of nerve thickening and anesthesia. Despite its bacterial origin and popular reputation, leprosy is minimally infectious, and isolation of affected persons is rarely justifiable.

TYPES OF SKIN INFECTIONS AND INFESTATIONS

As already noted, infectious agents of the skin include bacteria, viruses, fungi, and parasites. The following sections provide an overview of some of the more common types of skin infections and infestations that can occur in humans.

Among the best-known types of epidermal viral infections are herpes simplex (cold sores, fever blisters) and herpes zoster (shingles), which produce blisters within the epidermis. These viruses serve as useful examples in illustrating the importance of the immune system in defending against skin infections and infestations. The severity of infection with either of these viruses is influenced by the state of the person's immune system. Thus, they are more severe in injured persons, in the elderly, and in debilitated patients, especially those with cancer of the lymphoid system. Herpes zoster (shingles) and varicella (chickenpox) are caused by the same virus, and patients with shingles have previously had chickenpox.

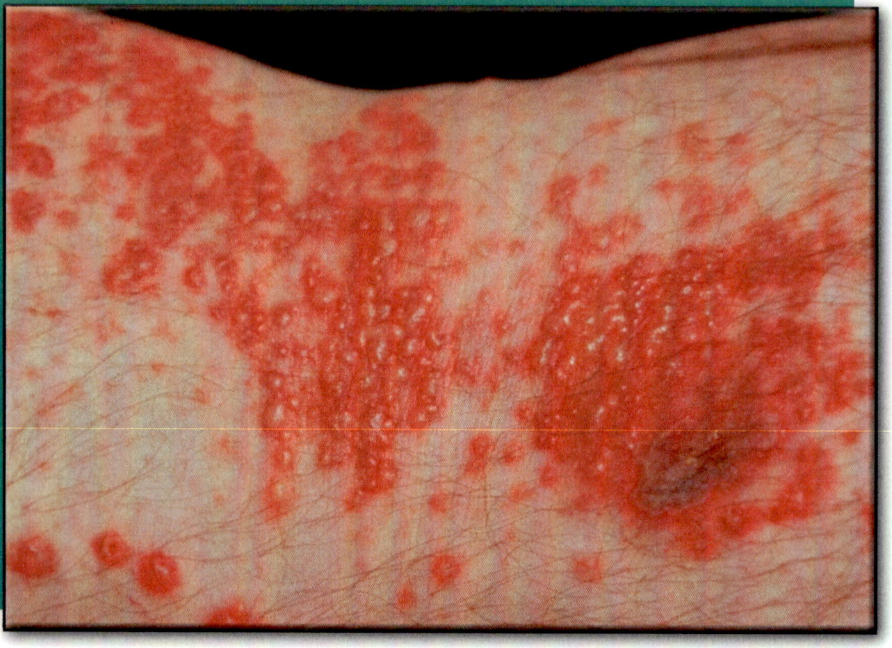

The virus that causes shingles can lay dormant for years before invading the skin, causing a painful, blistering rash. SIU/Visuals Unlimited/Getty Images

The virus remains dormant in the sensory nerves and is later reactivated, either spontaneously or following the impairment of immune defense mechanisms. The virus, by translocating along the nerve branches, invades the epidermis. The distribution of the ensuing vesicular rash, which is painful, is confined to the cutaneous distribution of the same sensory nerve.

Fungal infection is a common cause of chronic skin eruption. Several species of dermatophyte fungi may live on the dead horny layer of the skin. The inflammatory changes they produce are partly due to irritant products of the fungus, which diffuse into the skin, and partly to an immunologic reaction by the host in an attempt to eliminate the fungus. Yeasts, of which *Candida albicans* is the most common, are also a cause of chronic skin or mucous membrane infection. In patients receiving immunosuppressive drugs for organ transplantation, yeast infections may become systemic, and both yeast and dermatophyte infections may be extensive, persistent, and unresponsive to drug treatment. The availability of systemic antifungal drugs, including griseofulvin and the broad-spectrum imidazole group, has revolutionized the treatment of these disorders, but many patients with both minor and serious fungal infections remain resistant to drug treatment.

Skin infestations are frequent in persons living or working in overcrowded, unhygienic conditions. Pediculosis (crabs, lice, nits), which affects hairy areas, is diagnosed by identifying the egg capsules (nits) that are cemented to the hair shaft. Lice may also be visible near the base of the hair. Scalp, axillary, or pubic hair may be affected. Scabies, which is caused by a mite, is usually acquired through close personal contact, especially sexual contact. It affects all areas of the body except the soles of the feet, head, and neck (in infants these areas are also involved) and causes an itchy eruption that is largely an allergic reaction to the products of the mites. Chiggers, the larvae of certain mites, also live on humans and feed on blood. Their bite produces a wheal on the skin that is intensely itchy, the itchiness being caused by the digestive juices of the chiggers. Other bloodsucking insects that feed on humans are fleas, bedbugs, and ticks, which do not live on humans as primary hosts but in the ground, bedding, walls, and furniture. The more commonly seen lesions are those of the bedbug, which produces a burning wheal with a central punctured dot, and those of the flea, which produces a cluster of wheals and papules, resulting from the flea's habit of sampling several adjacent spots while feeding on the skin.

Abscess

An abscess is a localized collection of pus in a cavity formed from tissues that have been broken down by infectious bacteria. An abscess is caused when such bacteria as staphylococci or streptococci gain access to solid tissue (e.g., by means of a small wound on the skin). The toxins released by these multiplying bacteria destroy cells and thus trigger an acute inflammation at the site, with its characteristic signs of redness, pain, swelling, and heat. White blood cells (leukocytes) collect at the site. These leukocytes break down the dead tissues and absorb the bacteria by means of phagocytosis. Thick yellowish pus is formed from the broken-down tissues, the dead bacteria and leukocytes, and the extracellular fluid that has accumulated. At the same time, nearby healthy cells form a capsule of tissue around the pus and develop a cell wall that delimits the abscess from nearby healthy tissues. When the abscess is ruptured, either naturally or through medical intervention, the pus escapes, the swelling and pain are relieved, and the delimiting cell wall eventually grows back into the abscess cavity.

Abscesses may occur on the skin surface or within the body on such internal organs as the lungs, brain, kidneys, or tonsils. Treatment for those abscesses that do not naturally resolve themselves consists of cutting into the capsule and draining its pus contents. Antibiotics are also administered to help fight the infection. Antihistamines may be prescribed to reduce swelling. Care must be taken to prevent the pus and other infective contents from entering the bloodstream and thus being carried to surrounding tissues, where they can result in new abscesses.

Blastomycosis

Blastomycosis is an infection of the skin and viscera caused by fungal organisms of the genus *Blastomyces.* There are two major types of blastomycosis: the North American, caused by *B. dermatitidis*, and the South American, caused by *B. brasiliensis*. In North American blastomycosis, skin and lung lesions are most common: pulmonary lesions vary in size from granulomatous nodules to confluent, diffuse areas of pus-forming inflammation involving the entire lobe of the lung. In the skin, micro-abscesses lie just beneath the epidermis, the outermost layer of the skin, and are associated with a granulomatous appearance of the surrounding skin.

In South American blastomycosis, the portal of entry is usually the nasopharynx (the part of the alimentary canal between the cavity of the mouth and the esophagus that is continuous with the nasal passages); swelling and ulceration of the mouth or nose may cause the infection to spread to the nearby lymph nodes; primary lesions may also occur in the lymphoid tissues in the lower abdomen. In both North and South American varieties, the infection may spread not only to the lymph nodes but also to organs such as the brain, bones, liver, spleen, and adrenal glands. Treatment includes the use of antibiotics, antifungal agents, and sulfonamide drugs.

Erysipelas

Erysipelas is a contagious infection of the skin and underlying tissue, caused by group A B-hemolytic streptococcus bacteria. Erysipelas causes affected areas of skin to turn bright red and become slightly swollen. The swollen blotches have a distinct border and slowly expand into the surrounding skin. The lesions are most commonly seen on the face, scalp, hands, and legs. They feel hot to the touch and the patient is feverish.

Centuries ago erysipelas epidemics caused severe and often fatal infections. In 1089 CE one of the most severe epidemics was known as St. Anthony's fire because those who prayed to St. Anthony were said to recover; those who did not, died. Today erysipelas is a rather mild and relatively rare infection that clears up rapidly when penicillin or other antibiotics are taken. Even without treatment the infection usually disappears in several weeks, but treatment is necessary to ensure against such potential complications as nephritis, subcutaneous abscesses, and blood poisoning (septicemia) from bacterial toxins. Antibiotic treatment also ensures against a recurrence of the infection and its transmission to others.

Impetigo and Boils

Impetigo is an inflammatory skin infection that begins as a superficial blister or pustule that then ruptures and gives rise to a weeping spot on which the fluid dries to form a distinct honey-coloured crust. Impetigo is caused by *Staphylococcus* or *Streptococcus* bacteria. It is seldom contagious in adults, a little more so in children, and very contagious in newborn infants. Impetigo is the most common skin infection among children. It is spread by poor hygiene and crowding and is a particular problem in humid, hot weather. Impetigo is generally diagnosed by observation. In mild cases the lesions can be effectively treated with an antibiotic ointment; in more extensive involvement, especially in children, an oral antibiotic may be advisable.

A boil is an inflamed nodular swelling filled with pus, located at the site of a hair follicle. Boils are caused by

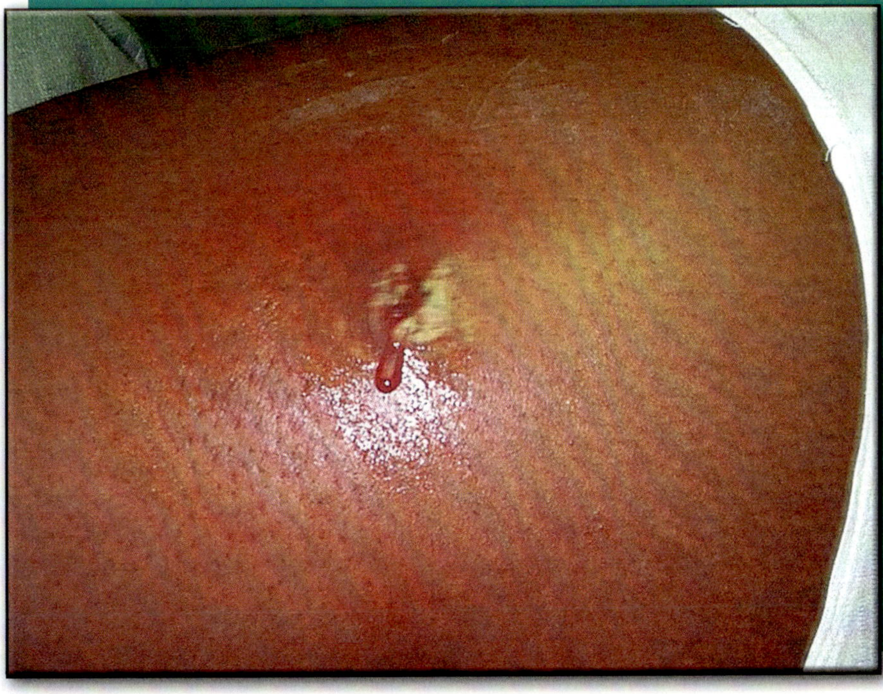

A draining boil that was caused by infection with methicillin-resistant Staphylococcus aureus *(MRSA) bacteria.* Bruno Coignard, M.D. and Jeff Hageman, M.H.S./CDC

staphylococcus organisms that infect the skin. The lesion is painful and feels hard to the touch. Healing begins after the pus is discharged. Boils are usually located in hairy body areas exposed to friction and maceration, such as the back of the neck, the face, armpits, buttocks, and groin. A sty is a boil located at the base of an eyelash. A carbuncle is an aggregation of adjoining boils with several centers of pus collection.

Existing skin disorders that lead to scratching may favour the entrance of the staphylococci into hair follicles, with resulting boil formation. Any general lowered state of health may also predispose individuals to furunculosis, although the condition also affects healthy people.

Some individuals seem more susceptible to boils than others, and in them the boils tend to recur. Ordinarily treatment is unnecessary, other than the use of measures to keep the affected area clean and protected from further infection. In more severe cases, antibiotics are usually effective. When boils occur in a patient at a hospital in which penicillin-resistant staphylococcal infections are endemic, they may constitute a serious medical problem, particularly when the patients are aged or debilitated.

A carbuncle is another type of inflammatory staphylococcal infection of the skin. A carbuncle typically consists of two or more interconnected boils called furuncles. These are painful red nodules that form yellowish heads which burst to release pus and dead tissue. Carbuncles, however, are larger than furuncles, generally involve deeper layers of the skin, and have multiple openings for the drainage of pus. They occur most often in hairy skin areas or areas that are subject to friction—e.g., the back of the neck, the armpits, and the buttocks.

While simple boils can be eliminated by the application of hot, moist dressings followed by washing with soap, carbuncles may have to be lanced and drained, a procedure that is often followed by antibiotic treatment. After the treatment, poor hygiene may lead to a recurrence.

Pediculosis

Pediculosis is the skin disorder caused by various species of bloodsucking lice that infect the scalp, groin, and body. The lice live on or close to the skin and attach their eggs to the hair or clothing of the host, on which they periodically feed. Their bite results in a small red spot that is extremely itchy and may become infected after repeated scratching.

Pinta

Pinta is a chronic tropical skin disease characterized initially by the appearance of dry, scaly papular lesions followed after several years by abnormally coloured patches called pintides. The pintides may be white, where pigment cells have been destroyed by the disease, or blue, red, or pink. The disease is native to Central and South America and is caused by infection with *Treponema carateum*, an organism that is indistinguishable from that of syphilis. There is some evidence of a degree of cross-immunity between the two diseases, and the treatment of both is the same. Unlike syphilis, however, pinta has little effect on the general health of the patient and is transmitted by nonvenereal contact.

Ringworm

Ringworm is characterized by superficial skin lesions that are caused by a highly specialized group of fungi called dermatophytes that live and multiply on the surface of the skin and feed on keratin. The fungi produce responses in the skin that vary from slight scaling to blistering and marked disruption of the keratin layer. The lesions are usually round or ring shaped and can be either dry and scaly or moist and covered with vesicles (blisters), depending on the body area and the type of fungus involved.

Ringworm is also referred to as tinea, both names referring to the round shape of most of the lesions, similar to the larva of the clothes moth, genus *Tinea*. In specifying the condition, *tinea* is usually followed by a modifying term indicating the body area or characteristics of the lesions. Thus, ringworm of the scalp, beard, and nails is also referred to as tinea capitis, tinea barbae or tinea

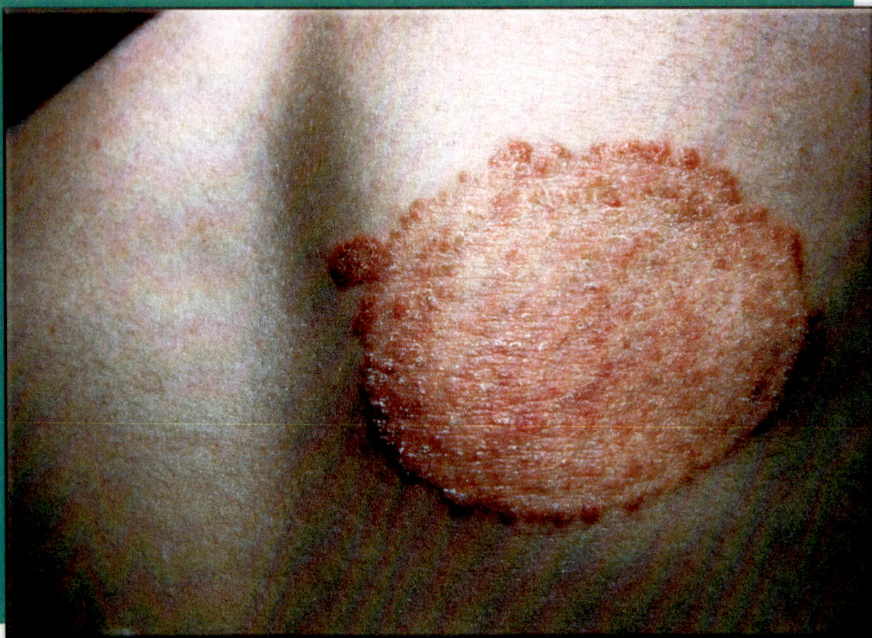

Ringworm is characterized by a red, scaly rash on the skin that forms in a decidedly circular or "ringlike" pattern. CMSP/Collection Mix: Subjects/ Getty Images

sycosis, and tinea unguium (also called onychomycosis), respectively; ringworm of the body, groin, hands, and feet, as tinea corporis, tinea cruris (also called jock itch), tinea manuum, and tinea pedis, respectively. Tinea pedis is commonly referred to as athlete's foot, which may be of either the dry or inflammatory type. In the latter type, the infection may lie dormant much of the time and undergo occasional acute exacerbations, with the development of vesicles (blisters) affecting chiefly the skin folds between the toes. The dry type is a chronic process marked by slight redness of the skin and dry scaling that may involve the sole and sides of the foot as well as the toenails, which become thick and brittle.

Varieties of ringworm characterized by specific skin lesions include: Oriental ringworm, Tokelau ringworm, or tinea imbricata (Latin: "overlapping like tiles"), so called because it occurs chiefly in tropical climates and consists of concentric rings of overlapping scales; crusted, or honeycomb, ringworm, also called favus, a ringworm of the scalp, characterized by the formation of yellow, cup-shaped crusts that enlarge to form honeycomb-like masses; and black dot ringworm, also a ringworm of the scalp, deriving its distinctive appearance and name from the breaking of the hairs at the scalp surface. Except for ringworm of the scalp, which tends to be highly contagious, the contraction of ringworm depends to a large extent on individual susceptibility and predisposing factors, such as excessive perspiration.

Diagnosis of ringworm is made by observation and by microscopic examination. Treatment with topical or oral antifungal agents may be effective. Limited exposure to ultraviolet radiation may also be helpful.

Scabies

Scabies, or sarcoptic itch, is a skin inflammation accompanied by severe nighttime itching caused by the itch mite (*Sarcoptes scabiei* var. *hominis*). The mite passes from person to person by close contact. Scabies is characteristically a disease of wartime, for living standards then drop, washing may be difficult, and people may be crowded together. The disease also afflicts many schoolchildren and residents of nursing homes, with periodic epidemics occurring even among persons with strict habits of hygiene and adequate living conditions.

Sarcoptes scabiei attains a length of about 0.35 mm (0.014 inch) and is barely visible to the unaided eye.

Despite its small size, it has quite formidable mouthparts and eight very powerful legs. With its hind legs, the female of the species hitches itself to the skin and, with its mouthparts thus closely applied to the skin, cuts its way down into the horny epithelial layer. The mite then tunnels horizontally and gouges out an easily recognizable burrow up to several inches long and usually not very straight. These burrows sometimes are visible as dark wavy lines. The female mite prefers the skin between the fingers and toes, on the wrist and elbows, in the armpits, below the breast, and on the male genitals. It does most of its moving at night. Sometimes it is visible at the far end of one of its burrows. The female mite lays eggs that hatch into larvae. The larvae emerge from the skin and molt several times through a nymph stage before they become adults and mate. The development from egg to laying adult frequently takes about three weeks.

The initial lesion produced by the burrowing mite becomes intensely itchy after a few days to about a month, and the scratching usually leads to secondary skin lesions consisting of papules (solid elevations), pustules, and crusted skin areas. In addition, a rash breaks out in parts of the body where there are no burrows—on the buttocks, over the shoulder blades, and on the abdomen. The cause of the rash is not clear; it is probably an allergic reaction to the presence of the mite on the body. It is intensely irritating and interferes with sleep.

Transmission of the mite is by skin-to-skin contact and by contamination of clothing or bedding. Transmission can be prevented by wearing clean underclothes and by frequently changing one's clothes and washing—conditions not always possible in time of war or mass migration. Effective treatment consists of covering the affected person from neck to feet with medicinal lotion that kills the mite. Several medications are available. One percent lindane lotion (gamma-benzene hexachloride) is effective but can be toxic. Permethrin, a synthetic drug based on chemicals derived from the chrysanthemum, is effective and quite safe, even in very young children. Sulfur-containing ointments may also work, but they are not well accepted for cosmetic reasons. It is desirable to treat an entire family or a group of people living together, for often the early burrowing stage of the disease causes no irritation, and a person can be infested without knowing it.

Warts

A wart, or verruca, is a well-defined growth of varying shape and size on the skin surface, caused by a virus. Essentially an infectious, benign skin tumour, a wart is composed of an abnormal proliferation of cells of the epidermis. The overproduction of these cells is caused by the viral infection. The most common type of wart is a round, raised lesion having a dry and rough surface. Flat or threadlike lesions are also seen. Warts are common and usually painless, except for those in pressure areas, such as the plantar warts occurring on the sole of the foot. They may occur as isolated lesions or grow profusely, especially in moist regions of the body surface. Genital warts, or condylomata acuminata, are wartlike growths in the pubic area that are accompanied by itching and discharge.

Warts have been studied at least since the time of Aulus Cornelius Celsus, the great Roman medical writer, in the 1st century CE, and they continue to interest researchers and challenge the therapeutic skills of experienced physicians. Warts are caused by a family of viruses known as human papillomaviruses, some of which have been shown to cause cervical cancer. A single wart may persist for many years without change, or it may spread and give rise to satellite warts in other parts of the body. Warts are considered contagious. Methods of treatment are many but are generally aimed at removing the wart with a minimum of scarring. These methods include the application of acids or other chemicals that gradually dissolve the wart, cryotherapy with liquid nitrogen, and, rarely, surgical excision, which remains the quickest procedure. Genital warts are sometimes treated with the application of podophyllin, a toxic substance derived from the mayapple. Warts sometimes disappear spontaneously.

CHAPTER 6

DISEASES AND DISORDERS OF SKIN TISSUES

Among the many noninfectious diseases and disorders of skin are skin allergies and inflammations, which range from dermatitis to hives and sunburn. In addition, there exist numerous localized skin conditions, such as excessive sweating, freckles, moles, and acne. While many of these localized conditions are benign, their conspicuous nature can be a source of anxiety for affected individuals. In some instances, however, a localized skin anomaly may serve as an indication of more serious disease. For example, a mole of irregular shape that enlarges over time may be a sign of melanoma, a cancerous disease of the skin.

SKIN ALLERGIES AND INFLAMMATIONS

Important examples of skin allergies and inflammations include dermatitis, hives, insect bites, and sunburn. Lesser-known conditions include chilblain, an abnormal sensitivity of the skin to cold, and pemphigus, the abnormal formation of large blisters on the skin surface. In many instances, these conditions are treated with anti-inflammatory agents, including creams applied to the skin and medications taken orally.

CHILBLAIN

Chilblain, also called pernio, or erythema pernio, is an inflammatory swelling of the skin of the hands or feet, resulting from exposure to cold. The condition is believed to result from cold hypersensitivity of small vessels of the skin. Tissue damage is less severe with chilblains than with frostbite, where the skin is actually frozen. Red, itching papules and patches of eroded tissue appear on the skin, which is cold and clammy to the touch. Severe chilblains may blister and swell. The condition is aggravated by warmth, and sudden rewarming is not recommended. The preferred treatment is to elevate the affected part and allow it to warm gradually at room temperature.

Dermatitis

Dermatitis, also called eczema, is an inflammation of the skin usually characterized by redness, swelling, blister formation, and oozing and almost always by itching. The term *eczema*, which formerly referred to the blistered, oozing state of inflamed skin, has by common usage come to have the same meaning as *dermatitis*.

Types of Dermatitis

Dermatitis may be classified into several types. Contact dermatitis results from contact of the skin with an irritating substance or a substance to which the person is allergic. The inflammation can result from contact with a strong acid or alkali or some other chemical, or it can result from contact with innocuous substances (e.g., cosmetics, soap, clothing) which are not primarily irritating in themselves but which produce a reaction in a person who has been sensitized by repeated exposure to them. The most common cause of contact dermatitis in the United States and some other countries is poison ivy. Many other plants can cause the condition. Chemical compounds that may cause contact dermatitis include such metals as nickel and chromium, certain aniline dyes, and many types of drugs. The prevention of contact dermatitis rests upon the identification of the particular irritant and subsequent avoidance of it.

Atopic dermatitis, the most common type of dermatitis, typically begins in infancy and can last into adulthood. It is characterized by redness, thickening, and scaling of the skin in patches, typically on the face, neck, hands, feet, in the crook of the elbow, or behind the knee. The skin becomes extremely dry, and this leads to itching. In adulthood the severity of skin symptoms tends to decrease. However, about three-quarters of affected individuals eventually develop hay fever or asthma. Scientists have identified abnormal levels of immune substances in people affected by atopic dermatitis, indicating that immune dysfunction plays an important role, likely triggering allergic reactions to normally innocuous substances. For example,

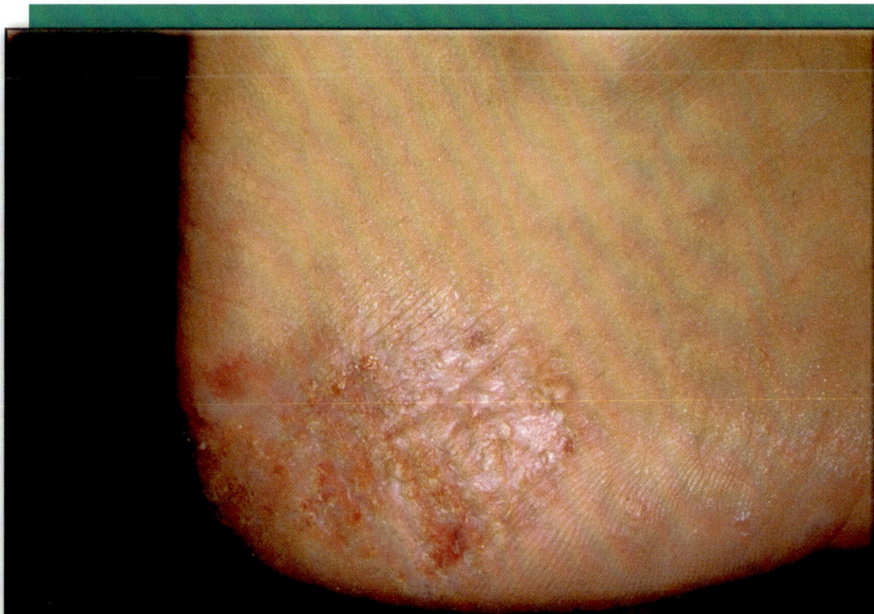

Also known as dermatitis, eczema is a skin condition that causes inflammation, rash, blisters, and, most prominently, itching. CMSP/Collection Mix: Subjects/Getty Images

in some affected people, chemical compounds associated with certain foods, plants, and animals may stimulate an inappropriate immune reaction that gives rise not only to skin symptoms but also to congestion, wheezing, and gastrointestinal upset. Irritants in tobacco smoke, detergents, industrial chemicals, and certain fabrics can also aggravate skin symptoms. The underlying cause of atopic dermatitis is not known, but it tends to run in families whose members have hay fever and asthma.

Stasis dermatitis is a skin inflammation affecting the ankles and lower legs. The condition is caused by chronic poor blood flow in the veins and particularly by varicose veins. The poor blood flow brings about swelling and a progressively more acute irritation of the skin that may lead to ulceration. Stasis dermatitis can be prevented if steps are taken early to improve the blood circulation of the legs, such as wearing supportive stockings or having surgery performed on the varicose veins.

Seborrheic dermatitis is a scaly skin condition that most frequently affects the scalp, dandruff being the common name for the skin particles that scale off the scalp. The condition generally involves body areas that are rich in sebaceous, or oil-secreting, glands, and it can also affect the forehead and eyebrows, the middle of the face, the area behind the ears, and the armpits. Most individuals with seborrheic dermatitis tend to have oily skin. During infancy, seborrheic dermatitis may commonly manifest itself as a yellowish scaling of part of the scalp, a condition referred to as cradle cap.

Neurodermatitis refers to a skin inflammation that is apparently caused by the patient's own repeated and chronic scratching of an itchy area of skin.

Exfoliative dermatitis is characterized by a generalized redness and scaling of the skin and usually arises as a complication of a preexisting skin disease or of an allergy.

Examples of such conditions include other types of dermatitis, such as contact or seborrheic dermatitis. More rarely, exfoliative dermatitis may be indicative of a systemic disease, such as cancer of the lymphoid tissue.

The onset of exfoliative dermatitis is gradual. Initial single lesions coalesce into large patches of scaly, red skin that may extend over any part of the body until no healthy skin is left. Hair and nails may lose their lustre and become brittle and fall. Occasionally, a yellow secretion may ooze out of the skin. Itching is variable and may be intense. The continuous shedding of the scales results in a significant loss of body protein. The maintenance of body temperature is also affected, because of the plugging of a majority of sweat ducts; the patient feels cold and feverish. Treatment focusses on the underlying primary disease. Rest and a high protein diet are beneficial. Exfoliative dermatitis is most common in middle life, affecting more men than women, by a ratio of about three to one.

Environmental Influences and Treatment

Research has indicated that environmental factors significantly influence the overall risk of dermatitis. For example, children who are breast-fed for four months or longer have a reduced risk of dermatitis. In addition, compounds called omega-3 fatty acids, which have anti-inflammatory properties, have become an important area of dermatitis research. Skin creams containing omega-3 fatty acids can lessen the severity of skin symptoms and, in some cases, prevent dermatitis. Studies comparing the early diets of children with and without dermatitis have indicated that incorporating fish into a child's diet before nine months of age reduces the risk of dermatitis by 25 percent. Scientists suspect that this reduction is mediated by omega-3 fatty acids, which are present in large amounts in some fish.

The general goals of treatment for dermatitis involve reducing symptoms, healing the skin, and preventing exposure to irritants and allergens that cause outbreaks. Special creams and lotions that contain anti-inflammatory compounds may be used to soften and soothe the skin, and topical corticosteroids may be applied to the skin to relieve itching. However, corticosteroid-containing medications can cause skin-thinning, dilation of superficial blood vessels that leads to unsightly red spots on the skin, and abnormal skin pigmentation. There is also a risk of systemic absorption of corticosteroids, which can lead to disruption of normal physiological steroid production. Topical immunomodulators (TIMs), which are steroid-free skin medications, have been developed. These agents work by inhibiting the activation of immune substances. However, due to their potentially dangerous side effects (e.g., lymphoma), TIMs are considered second-line treatments for dermatitis. Other therapies used include antihistamines, phototherapy, which uses ultraviolet radiation to suppress immune reactions, and photochemotherapy, which combines phototherapy with the administration of a light-sensitizing compound such as psoralen.

Hives

Hives, or urticaria, is a hypersensitive skin reaction characterized by the sudden appearance of very itchy, slightly raised, smooth, flat-topped wheals and plaques that are usually redder or paler than the surrounding skin. In the acute form, the skin lesions generally subside in 6 to 24 hours, but they may come and go and persist much longer in the chronic form.

Several specific causes of hives, as well as variant forms of its typical skin lesions, are denoted by qualifying the term *urticaria* with a descriptive word. Examples include urticaria bullosa, a rare type of allergic reaction characterized by the appearance of bullae or vesicles (large or small blisters); solar urticaria, produced by exposure to sunlight; and urticaria subcutanea, caused by swelling of the tissues underlying the skin.

Allergy to a specific food is probably the most frequent cause of acute urticaria. Fish, eggs, berries, and nuts head the list of common offenders. Hives may also be triggered by drugs, especially penicillin, by biologicals containing proteins, and by inhalants (e.g., pollens, insecticides, dust, feathers). Less frequently, physical agents, such as cold, heat, insect bites, and mechanical injury, as well as parasitic and other infectious diseases, may be triggers. Emotional and mental stresses are believed to be major and contributing causes of chronic urticaria.

The mechanism by which psychogenic factors give rise to chronic urticaria is not clear, but the overall sequence of biological events that triggers acute urticaria has been clarified. The mast cells lining the blood vessels contain histamine, which is released following contact of the mast cells with the irritating substance. Histamine in turn increases the permeability of the capillaries, so that plasma escapes into the spaces between the cells of the skin, giving rise to swellings that constitute the wheals and plaques. The itching is also thought to be caused by histamine.

Hives appear to show a familial incidence and are more common in persons with a history of allergic reactions. Treatment involves identification and subsequent avoidance of the allergen; administration of epinephrine and antihistamines may help to control the acute skin symptoms.

Insect Bite and Sting

A break in the skin caused by an insect and complicated by introduction into the skin of the insect's saliva, venom, or excretory products can lead to inflammation, sometimes with systemic complications. Specific components of these introduced substances are believed to give rise to an allergic reaction, which in turn produces skin lesions that may vary from a small itching wheal, or slightly elevated area of the skin, to large areas of inflamed skin covered by vesicles and crusted lesions.

Flying insects, such as flies, gnats, and mosquitoes, attack exposed body parts, each bite resulting in a single itchy wheal that generally subsides within hours. Crawling insects may reach any part of the body, including the covered areas, and are more likely to remain there, generating skin diseases characteristic of each insect.

Stinging insects produce a painful swelling of the skin, the severity of the lesion varying according to the location of the sting and the identity of the insect. Many species of bees and wasps have two poison glands, one gland secreting a toxin in which formic acid is one recognized constituent, and the other secreting an alkaline neurotoxin; acting independently, each toxin is rather mild, but when they are injected together through the stinger, the combination has strong irritating properties. In a small number of cases the second occasion of a bee or wasp sting causes a severe allergic reaction known as anaphylaxis.

Hornets, some ants, centipedes, scorpions, and spiders also sting. Some insects leave their stinger in the wound. Multiple stings may give rise to severe systemic symptoms and in rare instances may even lead to death. The bites of some spiders are known to be lethal, particularly to young children.

Pemphigus

Pemphigus is a group of skin diseases characterized by large blisters that appear on the skin and mucous membranes.

Pemphigus diseases include pemphigus vulgaris, pemphigus vegetans, pemphigus foliaceus, pemphigus erythematosus, and benign familial pemphigus.

The most common and most severe of these diseases is pemphigus vulgaris, in which large, flaccid blisters erupt on otherwise healthy-looking skin and mucous membranes. The first site of blistering is often the mouth. The blisters rupture easily, leaving weeping, encrusted areas that do not heal. Pain from mouth lesions can prevent the individual from eating. If untreated, the disease can cause fluid and electrolyte imbalance, sepsis, and death. Pemphigus vegetans is similar. Both are autoimmune diseases caused by antibodies that are produced against proteins (antigens) found within cells of the outermost

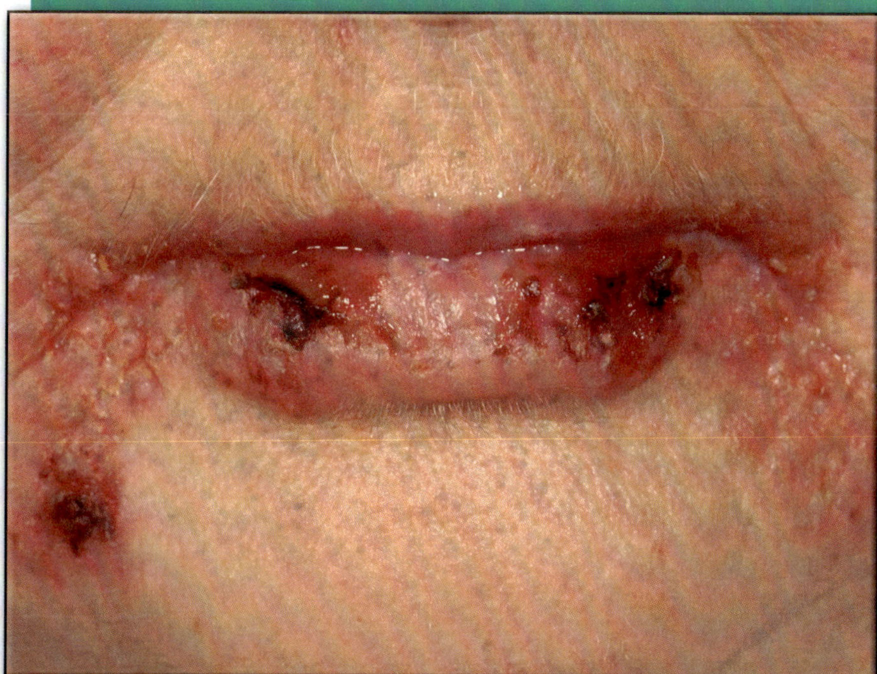

Mouth sores typical of pemphigus vegetans, one of the more serious forms of the autoimmune disease pemphigus. Biophoto Associates/Photo Researchers, Inc.

layer of the skin, called the epidermis. The interaction between autoantibodies and these antigens results in a loss of cohesion among skin cells and the degeneration of skin layers. The clefts and splits within the degenerating skin layers fill with fluid, leading to the characteristic blistering. These diseases can be successfully treated with immunosuppressive drugs and high doses of systemic corticosteroids.

Pemphigus foliaceus and pemphigus erythematosus are less severe. Mucous membranes are rarely involved. Lesions may be found on the scalp, face, or trunk, or they may spread. They also arise from an autoimmune reaction, but the process usually occurs nearer the surface of the epidermis. Low doses of systemic steroids usually control them.

Benign familial pemphigus, also called Hailey-Hailey disease, is an inherited disorder characterized by blisters on the neck, groin, and armpits. Unlike other forms of pemphigus, autoantibodies are not apparent. Topical and systemic antibiotics are used to treat flare-ups.

Psoriasis

Psoriasis is a chronic, recurrent inflammatory skin disorder. The most common type, called plaque psoriasis (psoriasis vulgaris), is characterized by reddish, slightly elevated patches or papules (solid elevations) covered with silvery-white scales. In most cases, the lesions tend to be symmetrically distributed on the elbows and knees, scalp, chest, and buttocks. The lesions may remain small and solitary or coalesce into large plaques that often form geometrical patterns with a central area of normal skin. In many cases the nails become thickened, irregularly laminated, and brittle. In addition to plaque psoriasis, there are four other types of psoriasis, including guttate, pustular, inverse (or flexular), and erythrodermic.

Psoriasis is an immune-mediated (or autoimmune) disorder that occurs when immune cells known as T lymphocytes, or T cells, attack healthy skin cells in both the nonvascular horny outer layer of the skin and its deeper vascular layer. This attack causes the life span of the skin cells to shorten to about 3 to 5 days (skin cells normally live about 20 to 28 days) and forces the cells to reproduce more rapidly than normal. Psoriasis occurs in both sexes with equal frequency, being most prevalent between the ages of 10 and 30. It is most often seen in northern climates. An estimated 2 to 3 percent of the U.S. population is affected by psoriasis. In contrast, between 0.05 and 0.3 percent of Asians experience the condition. In European countries the incidence of psoriasis is highly variable, affecting anywhere from less than 1 percent to more than 6 percent of populations.

The onset of psoriasis is usually gradual but occasionally explosive. Precipitating factors may include injury to the skin, acute infection, and psychological upsets. Ordinarily, the lesions become less severe and sometimes disappear during the summer, possibly owing to the effect of sunlight. The severe complications of psoriasis are extensive sloughing of the outer layer of the skin, with resulting inflammation, and psoriatic arthritis. Generally, however, individuals with psoriasis are in relatively good health. The variability in the progression and severity of the disorder has led researchers to suspect that the underlying causes of psoriasis are the result of complex interactions between genetic and environmental factors.

There is no permanent cure for psoriasis, but there are a variety of treatments aimed at relieving the associated skin symptoms. Topical treatments for psoriasis come in different forms (e.g., creams and gels) and generally provide relief from inflammation and scaling. Some, such as retinoids (derivatives of vitamin A) and synthetic forms of vitamin D, work by slowing skin cell reproduction, whereas others, such as corticosteroids, coal-tar ointment, and salicylic acid, work by reducing inflammation. Psoriasis can also be treated with phototherapy, in which the skin is exposed to ultraviolet light. While phototherapy can be highly effective, it does have side effects, including pain, irregular pigmentation, and scarring. In addition, long-term treatments are associated with an increased risk of skin cancer. Oral medications are also available to treat psoriasis but are often used as a last resort. This is because the drugs that are most effective in treating psoriasis suppress the immune system, making patients susceptible to a multitude of infections and illnesses that can be life-threatening. Oral drugs that are used to reduce inflammation include methotrexate, cyclosporine, and azathioprine. Oral drugs called biologics (because they are made from human or animal proteins) modulate the immune system by attacking immune cells that are working improperly. Several biologics have been approved for psoriasis, including alefacept (Amevive), infliximab (Remicade), and etanercept (Enbrel).

Sunburn

Sunburn is an acute cutaneous inflammation caused by overexposure to ultraviolet (UV) radiation of the so-called UVB wavelength band (290–320 nanometres; a nanometre is 10^{-9} metre), which originates from sunlight or artificial sources. Reactions to overexposure range in severity from mild redness and tenderness to intense pain, edema (swelling), and blistering. Systemic symptoms include shock, chills, fever, and nausea. The visible manifestations of sunburn usually begin within 6–12 hours after the first ultraviolet exposure and peak within 24–28 hours, followed by a gradual easing of symptoms and light tanning or "peeling" (the sloughing off of the skin), depending on the severity of the burn.

Sunburn begins within 15 minutes after exposure to UV rays, triggering inflammation (the erythema, or redness). To limit epidermal damage, the pigment melanin (which is produced by epidermal cells called melanocytes) darkens through oxidation. Melanocytes increase in both size and number within two to three days, producing more melanin. Within days, a protective tan (in mild cases of sunburn) is formed.

Cold compresses applied to the affected skin and analgesic medicines can relieve some of the pain of sunburn. Severe sunburn can be prevented by limiting exposure to ultraviolet rays until a sufficient protective tan has developed or by applying a sunscreen that contains either para-aminobenzoic acid (PABA) or benzophenones. Scientists are developing UV-sensitive devices that warn of potential overexposure to sunlight in order to prevent sunburn. These devices, which could be worn around the wrist, indicate the increasing risk of erythema by using simple colour changes that are induced by UV rays. A long-term effect of prolonged and repeated exposure to sunlight can cause a number of skin disorders, including basal-cell carcinomas (small, smooth nodules) that usually appear on the face.

LOCALIZED SKIN CONDITIONS

Localized skin conditions are so called because they are superficially restricted to a specific region or area of skin. Birthmarks, moles, and freckles are examples. In addition, certain disorders of hair follicles and sweat glands are considered localized skin diseases. Examples include local hyperhidrosis (excessive sweating) and miliaria, in which lesions form at the sites of sweat pores. Some of these conditions, although localized superficially on the skin, are hereditary and may be associated with physiological affects that are more systemic in nature.

Abnormalities in Pigmentation

An increase in melanin pigmentation may be caused by an increased density of melanocytes, by abnormal packaging of melanin, or by increased melanin production. Pigmented birthmarks usually reflect local increases in melanocyte numbers, but in certain rare congenital pigmentary disorders, such as von Recklinghausen neurofibromatosis, there is abnormal packaging of melanin within the melanocytes. Pigment production in the skin is regulated by a pituitary peptide hormone, melanocyte-stimulating hormone, and the increase in melanin pigmentation seen with pituitary tumours may reflect overproduction of this hormone by the pituitary.

Both suntans and postinflammatory pigmentation result from the overproduction of melanin by melanocytes. In suntans melanin overproduction occurs in response to ultraviolet light and protects the skin against sunburn and the carcinogenic actions of ultraviolet rays. Postinflammatory pigmentation follows a number of inflammatory skin disorders, including chronic dermatitis, acne vulgaris, lichen planus, and drug reactions. It is more common in dark-skinned than in fair-skinned persons. In suntans and postinflammatory pigmentation there is usually no increase in the number of melanocytes.

Loss of melanin pigmentation may be caused by the absence of melanocytes, as in vitiligo; reduced or absent synthesis of melanin by melanocytes, as in albinism and phenylketonuria; abnormal packaging of melanin in melanosomes, as in the Chediak-Higashi syndrome; or insufficient transfer of melanosomes to keratinocytes, as

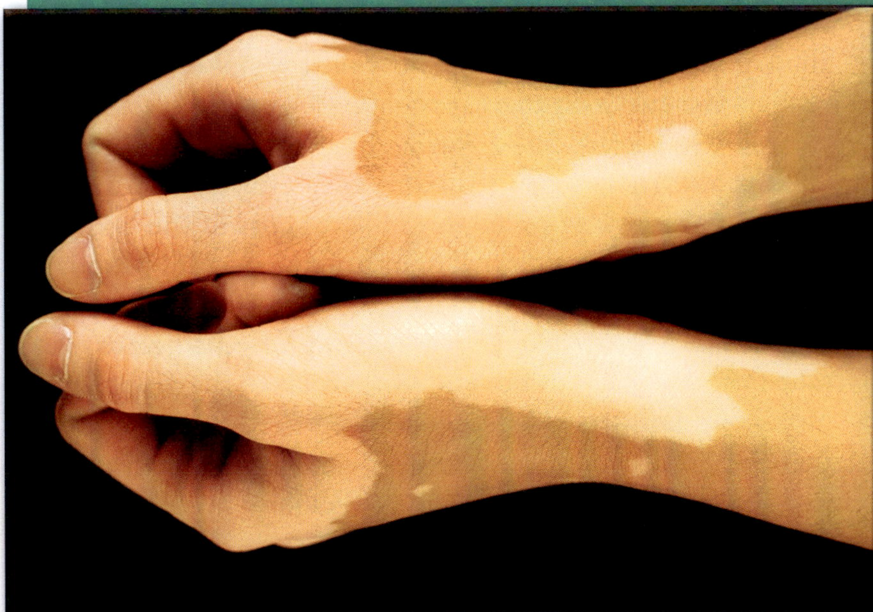

Woman displaying vitiligo (also known as leukoderma) on her hands and wrists. This common condition occurs when there is some kind of dysfunction of melanocytes, the cells that create pigment. CMSP/Collection Mix: Subjects/Getty Images

in hypopigmentation secondary to atopic dermatitis or psoriasis.

Vitiligo, also called leukoderma, is a common hereditary disorder of pigmentation that results in the widespread appearance of depigmented patches, notably around the mouth, anogenital area, eyelids, elbows, knees, and backs of the hands, due to an absence of melanocytes in these areas. Though the pigment-making cells of the skin, or melanocytes, are structurally intact, they have lost the ability to synthesize the pigment. The reason for this condition is unclear. Vitiligo appears clinically as milk-white, irregularly oval patches of skin, which are small at the beginning but enlarge gradually. These patches are roughly symmetrical. The hair growing in the depigmented area is also white. Individuals with vitiligo (about 1 percent of the adult population) are usually in good general health, but vitiligo presents a cosmetic problem that can be serious in dark-skinned individuals. Vitiligo is usually a slowly progressive disorder that is probably the result of abnormal immunologic reactions against constituents of the body's own cells (autoimmunity). The normal skin colour rarely returns and there is no known cure.

Certain chemicals found in plants, the psoralens, if taken orally or applied to the skin enhance the ability of ultraviolet light to induce pigmentation. Although rarely successful, treatment with psoralens and ultraviolet radiation has restored pigmentation. Persons with vitiligo should avoid sunlight, which accentuates the contrast between normal and depigmented skin.

Freckles

Freckles, or ephelides, are small, brownish, well-circumscribed, stainlike spots on the skin occurring most frequently in red- or sandy-haired individuals. In genetically predisposed individuals who have been exposed to the ultraviolet radiation of sunlight, production of the pigment melanin increases in the pigment cells of the skin (melanocytes). The number of melanocytes does not increase. Freckles do not form on surfaces that have not been exposed to the sun. The freckles usually appear after the age of five and tend to fade somewhat in adults. Apart from avoiding sunlight, there is no known way of preventing them. They may, on occasion, be confused with pigmented nevi.

Moles

Moles are pigmented, flat or fleshy skin lesions and are composed for the most part of an aggregation of melanocytes. In thicker moles, nerve elements and connective tissue are also present. Moles vary in colour from light to dark brown or black. When deposition of melanin occurs in the dermis, the deeper layer of the skin located underneath the epidermis, the lesion has a bluish cast. Moles may be present at birth. More frequently, however, they appear and evolve in character during childhood.

A new mole is usually flat and of the junctional type (junction nevus), so called because it is located between the dermis and the epidermis. It sometimes remains there, in which case the possibility of malignant development is increased. In most instances, however, the original mole evolves into a slightly raised lesion located in the dermis (intradermal nevus). Examination of the tissue of an actively changing mole in a child may show transformations resembling cancer, but actually such lesions are benign. Malignant melanoma is almost never seen until after puberty. During pregnancy, existing moles may enlarge and new ones may appear. Moles will sometimes disappear with age.

Nevi

Nevi (singular *nevus*) are congenital skin lesions, or birthmarks, caused by abnormal pigmentation or by proliferation of blood vessels and other dermal or epidermal structures. Nevi may be raised or may spread along the surface of the skin. In other types, such as the blue nevus, proliferative tissue is buried deep within the dermis, the lower layer of the skin.

Most types of nevi are formed by the overgrowth of normal skin components that retain their usual functions. Some nevi, however, are precancerous and lose their normal organization when they become malignant. Premalignant nevi include the sebaceous nevus, a congenital formation containing hair follicles and sebaceous glands, and the giant pigmented, or bathing trunk, nevus, a large, irregular, dark brown or black patch associated with malignant melanoma. Some pigmented nevi, such as the blue nevus and the junctional nevus, may be associated with skin cancers but are not widely considered precancerous. Other pigmented nevi may be associated with systemic diseases. Café-au-lait spots, light brown spots that can occur anywhere on the body, occur naturally in 10 percent of the white population but may also be a symptom of Albright disease. Mongolian spot, a blue-black patch on the lower back, occurs in 90 percent of American Indian, black, and Asiatic persons.

Although pigmented nevi are among the most common of these skin growths, other varieties of nevus are also known. Vascular nevi, or hemangiomas, produce the familiar "port wine stain" birthmark. They are composed of blood vessels and often resolve themselves with time. Epidermal nevi, of which the sebaceous nevus is an example, develop from the proliferation of normal epidermal tissues and are usually flesh-coloured or yellowish.

Skin Blood Vessel Disorders

Blood circulation in the skin serves both to supply nutrients and as a means of regulating temperature. The structural and functional organization of the skin's vascular system is complex, and there are major regional variations. Skin blood vessel disorders may arise from an increase in the viscosity of blood contents or from abnormalities of the vessels themselves. Increased viscosity may be due to an overabundance of red blood cells (polycythemia) or an increase in one or more fractions of the protein content of the plasma. Hyperglobulinemia is an example of the latter. In functional disorders of the blood vessels, nervous control of the vessels may be disturbed, leading to vascular spasm or dilatation (flushing). In Raynaud phenomenon, the vascular spasm is severe, affecting the extremities and leading to attacks of cold, white fingers. Milder degrees of spasm, as well as increases in blood viscosity, may cause a purple discoloration of the skin (cyanosis), which may assume a reticulate pattern (livedo reticularis).

Damage to the vessel walls themselves may perturb skin circulation. Causes include atherosclerosis resulting from age-related degenerative changes, disturbance of lipid (fat) metabolism, and inflammation of the vessel wall. When disease of the blood vessels is severe, lack of blood in the affected areas may cause skin ulcers. Chilblains occur when the skin is persistently chilled, leading to protracted vessel spasm, cyanosis, coldness, and ultimately ulceration of the affected area.

Diseases of Hair and Pilosebaceous Follicles

Hair is of little functional value in humans. Many systemic diseases, however, alter the appearance and growth patterns of hair. In diseases of malnutrition, such as kwashiorkor, the scalp hair becomes reddish brown, sparse, and brittle. Acute protein starvation may lead to the cessation of hair growth and constriction of the hair shafts. Chronic iron deficiency may cause diffuse hair loss (alopecia). Since the continuous hair growth of healthy persons involves the cells of the hair root in exuberant mitotic activity, hair is especially vulnerable to the cytotoxic action of drugs. Acute hair loss is an early side effect of the cytotoxic drugs used in cancer chemotherapy.

Acute diffuse hair loss (telogen effluvium) may also occur after severe fevers and childbirth. It appears to be caused by an abrupt reduction in the proportion of actively growing hairs, and after a few months the hair regrows normally without treatment. The hair follicles may become inflamed, forming small pustules, which, in severe cases, result in bald, scarred areas with destroyed follicles.

Both pattern baldness in men and hirsutism in women are thought to be under the control of the steroid sex hormones. Male pattern baldness occurs to some extent in almost all men. It may start any time after puberty and is distinguished from other forms of alopecia by the pattern of frontal and temporal hair recession and thinning over the crown. On the affected areas of the scalp a downy hair called vellus replaces the former long, sturdy, pigmented terminal hair. Almost as common is the reverse process, in which hair that was formerly vellus alters to the long pigmented terminal type and becomes more visible. When this occurs in the areas of the female body sensitive to male sex hormones, and especially when it follows the adult male pattern of hair distribution, it is known as hirsutism. Some affected women have endocrinologic abnormalities, including ovarian cystic disease or overactive adrenal glands, that elevate the levels of androgen (male sex hormones). These women may also have menstrual irregularities or be infertile. Hormonal treatment or, in less extensively hirsute women, electrolytic depilation may be helpful.

Among persons with curly hair, and especially among blacks, cut ends of hair may curve and bury themselves in the skin, causing acute pustular reactions. These ingrowing hairs, or pili incarnati, affect 70 percent of black men who are clean-shaven.

Acne

Acne is any inflammatory disease of the sebaceous, or oil, glands of the skin. There are some 50 different types of acne. In common usage, the term *acne* is frequently used alone to designate acne vulgaris, or common acne, probably the most prevalent of all chronic skin disorders.

Acne vulgaris results from an interplay of heredity factors, hormones, and bacteria. In susceptible individuals, it begins in the teen years, being caused by overactive sebaceous glands, which are stimulated by the upsurge in the circulating level of male sex hormones that accompanies the onset of puberty. The primary lesion of acne vulgaris is the comedo, or blackhead, which consists of a plug of sebum (the fatty substance secreted by a sebaceous gland), cell debris, and microorganisms (especially the bacterium *Propionibacterium acnes*) filling up a hair follicle. Comedones may be open, their upper or visible portion being darkened by oxidative changes, or they may be closed (i.e., not reaching the surface to be extruded), in which case, they may be starting points for pustules and deep inflammatory lesions.

The severity of acne is divided generally into four grades. In grade I, comedones may be sparse or profuse but there is little or no inflammation. In grade II, comedones are intermingled with superficial pustules and papules (small, solid, usually conical elevations). The lesions are ordinarily confined to the face and do not produce significant scarring, unless there has been continued scratching and picking. At this stage, topical (locally applied) medication is reasonably effective. Complete spontaneous remission is ordinarily seen within one to two years. In grades III and IV, the acne is characterized by comedones and pustules and deeper inflamed nodules, which are thought to result from the rupture of the sebaceous duct, with extrusion of sebum and bacterial products into the skin tissue. The lesions are likely to extend from the face to the neck and upper trunk and to produce a permanent scarring of the skin.

The course of acne vulgaris is variable, persistence being ordinarily directly related to the severity of the lesions, although changes of climate and emotional stress may markedly improve or exacerbate the acne lesions. Methods of treatment vary from topical medication to sunlight and ultraviolet light, antibiotics, and hormones. In a high proportion of cases, however, the tendency is toward spontaneous cure over several months.

Diseases of Sweat Glands

Most sweat glands in humans are eccrine (i.e., they secrete outwardly) and are under the control of the autonomic nervous system. Eccrine sweat glands are distributed uniformly over the body and function mainly in controlling temperature, although on the hands and feet they assist grip. Inability to secrete adequate sweat (anhidrosis) is usually a congenital abnormality.

Most serious disorders of the eccrine sweat glands result from the retention of sweat. Prickly heat (miliaria) occurs in persons living in a hot, humid environment and is due to sweat retention brought on by the combination of increased sweat production and blockage of the duct from hydration of the surrounding horny layer of skin. The gland continues to secrete, and the pressure may rupture the sweat duct at its junction with the epidermis. In heatstroke, another disorder of the eccrine sweat glands, the glands are exhausted and unable to secrete sweat. Hyperpyrexia, an excessive rise in body temperature, may ensue and is sometimes fatal. The most common disorder of the eccrine glands, however, is hyperhidrosis, or excessive sweating, of the palms, soles, armpits, and face.

Apocrine sweat glands, which are normally limited to the armpits, perineum, and genitalia, differ anatomically and physiologically from eccrine sweat glands. In the apocrine glands the secretions are concentrated at the free end of the cell, which is cast off along with the secretory products. Apocrine secretion is oily, opalescent, and odourless when secreted, but acquires an offensive smell when it mingles with the bacteria of the skin. The actions of deodorants and antiperspirants are based mainly on an antibacterial effect, on mechanical blockade of the apocrine gland pores, or both.

Hyperhidrosis

Hyperhidrosis, also spelled hyperidrosis, may be either general or local. A person may sweat profusely in the armpits and on the palms, soles, and forehead when excited, afraid, or anxious. Emotional stress normally stimulates sweating in these areas, but in hyperhidrosis excessive sweating may follow minor stimuli or no obvious stimulus at all. Hyperhidrosis may be an occupational problem for those who handle books, papers, or metallic objects that can rust.

Inflammation of the sympathetic nerves can also cause local hyperhidrosis, as can trench or immersion foot (resulting from long periods when the feet are soaked and cold) and encephalitis. Generalized sweating can occur after a fever or when a person is overheated or has taken aspirin, alcohol, or a hot drink. Heavy general sweating may accompany malaria, typhoid fever, tuberculosis, brucellosis, diabetes mellitus, or hyperthyroidism. Encephalitis and diencephalic epilepsy can also cause this type of sweating.

Ichthyosis

Ichthyosis, also known as fish-skin disease, is a group of conditions involving dryness and scaliness of the skin. Ichthyoses usually are hereditary, although some forms may be acquired. The conditions range from mild skin dryness (xeroderma) to severe dryness and thickening of the skin with the formation of skin "plates" separated by fissures (harlequin ichthyosis).

Icthyoses are brought about by excessive growth of the horny outermost covering of the skin. The dead cells of this horny layer do not slough off at the normal rate but tend instead to adhere to the skin surface to form scales. Horny plaques and papules may also be present in more severe cases. The skin in this condition is intolerant of even the mildest irritants and is prone to severe chapping and fissuring in cold weather. With the exception of harlequin ichthyosis, which is visible in newborns, ichthyosis is usually not detected at birth. However, as the child grows older, dry branny scaling will appear, being most marked on the extensor surfaces of the extremities.

Ichthyosis may sometimes be associated with a deficiency of the sweat glands and, less frequently, with irregularities in the growth of hair, teeth, and nails. In its mild and simplest form, ichthyosis is probably the most common of the hereditary skin disturbances.

Miliaria

Miliaria is an inflammatory disorder of human skin that is characterized by multiple small lesions at the site of sweat pores. It is brought about by the blockage of sweat ducts and the resulting escape of sweat into various levels of the skin. Most cases of miliaria occur in extremely hot weather. The lesions tend to disappear with cooler weather and the resultant decrease in sweating. There are four varieties of miliaria.

In miliaria crystallina, the sweat escapes into the superficial region of the epidermis, the outermost horny layer of the skin, where it collects in tiny, clear, noninflammatory, dewdrop vesicles (blisters). These are most commonly seen in patients with fever or after a sunburn.

Miliaria rubra, or prickly heat, the most common form of sweat retention, results from the escape of sweat into the epidermis, where it produces discrete, densely packed, pinhead vesicles or red papules (solid, usually conical elevations). These lesions occur chiefly on the trunk and extremities, where they cause itching and burning. The incidence of prickly heat is highest in tropical climates, where it most commonly affects infants.

In miliaria pustulosa, there are pustules, or small elevations of the skin filled with pus, at the site of sweat retention.

Miliaria profunda is a deep type of sweat retention, the sweat escaping into the dermis, the vascular layer of the skin located below the epidermis. The lesions, in this form of miliaria, are firm papules.

Nail Disease

The most common causes of diseased nails are chronic paronychia—infection of the soft tissue of the fingers between the lateral edges of the nail plates and the lateral nail folds—fungus infections, trauma, psoriasis, impaired circulation, and dermatitis. Chronic paronychia is an occupational hazard of dishwashers, bar workers, hairdressers, and vegetable preparers. When the cuticle is lost, water, bacteria, and yeasts seep under the nail fold and cause inflammation. The lateral nail folds extrude beads of pus when they are squeezed. The infection is commonly caused by the yeast *Candida albicans,* and when this organism is identified, infection elsewhere in the body should be sought.

Like the hair, the nails may be useful indicators of skin diseases and of internal disorders. Psoriasis causes pitting on the surface of the nails and an increase in their growth rate. Lichen planus causes a characteristic scarring of the posterior nail fold, leading to fusion of the posterior nail fold with the nail plate. Club-shaped deformity of the nail plate is associated with chronic chest disease and cyanotic congenital heart disease. A reduction in the rate of nail growth, a yellow discoloration of the nail plate, and a smooth curvature to the nails are all features of the yellow nails syndrome, a rare hereditary condition in which the lymphatic drainage system of the body is defective. In chronic anemia the nail plate may become concave (koilonychia).

Transverse depressions of the nail plates called Beau's lines result from temporary interruption of nail growth and are seen in a number of acute illnesses, including coronary thrombosis, pneumonia, and severe injuries. Various forms of interference with the blood supply may affect the nail matrix and produce irregular growth of the nails. Drug treatment may cause shedding of the nails. Photo-onycholysis—destruction of the nails from exposure to sunlight—occurs in patients taking photosensitizing drugs such as certain broad-spectrum antibiotics.

CHAPTER 7

DISEASES AND DISORDERS OF CONNECTIVE TISSUE

Diseases of connective tissue may affect the tissue's primary structure or may be maladies in which the connective tissues are the site of several more or less distinctive immunological and inflammatory reactions. Among the latter are many widely recognized conditions, including rheumatoid arthritis, systemic lupus erythematosus, rheumatic fever, and osteoarthritis. In many instances, the underlying causes of immunological and inflammatory reactions involving connective tissues are unknown. It is suspected, however, that both genetic and environmental factors contribute to these conditions.

FEATURES OF CONNECTIVE TISSUE DISEASE

Acquired connective tissue diseases display certain common clinical features, including inflammation of the joints (polyarthralgia and arthritis), serous (fluid-exuding) membranes (pleurisy and pericarditis), and small blood vessels (vasculitis) and a high frequency of involvement of various internal organs that are particularly rich in connective tissue (e.g., the lungs). The walls of inflamed blood vessels, portions of which may become necrotic (i.e., may die), are often found to contain characteristic deposits of hyaline (translucent) material called fibrinoid because staining with dyes (e.g., eosin) reveals tinctorial properties similar to fibrin (a fibrous protein that forms the lattice of blood clots).

A number of observations suggest that acquired connective tissue diseases are autoimmune diseases—i.e., diseases that result from reactions against components of the body as if they were foreign substances. In general terms these observations are that: (1) there are abnormally high levels of immunoglobulins in the blood; the immunoglobulins, also called gamma globulins, consist wholly or chiefly of antibodies; (2) these antibodies include several directed against particular serum proteins and other components of the affected person's own tissues; (3) there are complexes (combinations) of these antibodies and their antigens at the sites of tissue damage; (4) at the sites of tissue damage there are also aggregations of the cells (plasma cells and lymphocytes) that are responsible for the production of antibodies; (5) there is a favourable response to treatment with medications, such as corticosteroid hormones, known or believed to inhibit the production of antibodies; (6) connective tissue diseases are associated with other disorders known or suspected to be the result of an aberrant immune system.

Antibody-antigen interactions may result in the destruction of red or white blood cells or platelets or may inactivate circulating hormones or enzymes. The antibody-antigen complexes may be deposited in the walls of blood vessels and there combine with a substance in the blood called complement, with a variety of injurious effects, including those seen in serum sickness and in rheumatoid arthritis and the kidney damage seen in systemic lupus erythematosus. Last, the interaction may result in cellular immunity, which plays an important role in certain autoimmune disorders that involve solid organs, as well as in transplant rejection and cancer immunity.

DISORDERS OF INFLAMMATION AND AUTOIMMUNITY

There are many different disorders of inflammation and autoimmunity that can compromise the structure and function of connective tissue. Well-known disorders, as mentioned previously, include rheumatoid arthritis, systemic lupus erythematosus, and rheumatic fever. Other important disorders include amyloidosis, scleroderma, and Sjögren syndrome. Because the underlying causes of these conditions frequently are unknown, treatment, rather than being curative, is often aimed at controlling symptoms.

Amyloidosis

Amyloidosis is a disease characterized by the deposition of an abnormal protein called amyloid in the connective tissues and organs of the body that inhibits normal functioning. Amyloid is a fibrous, insoluble protein-carbohydrate complex that forms when normally soluble proteins such as antibodies become misfolded and adopt a fibril structure. There are different types of amyloid, and each type can be distinguished by the major protein component that it contains.

Amyloidosis may be systemic (affecting tissues and organs throughout the body), or it may be localized in tumourlike masses within certain organs. The organs most commonly affected by the disease include the kidneys, heart, liver, spleen, lungs, and skin. Symptoms vary depending on which organ or organs are affected. For example, symptoms of intestinal bleeding, malnutrition, constipation, and diarrhea may be associated with amyloid deposits in the gastrointestinal tract, whereas symptoms of shortness of breath and heart failure may be associated with amyloid deposits in the heart.

There are different types of amyloidosis, which can be classified as primary, secondary, or hereditary. Primary systemic amyloidosis is rare and occurs in the absence of underlying disease. Symptoms typically appear in the fifth or sixth decade of life and may include skin abnormalities (e.g., discoloration and nodule formation), heart failure, kidney failure, and enlargement of the spleen and liver. Though the cause of this form is unknown, it is associated with the abnormal production of antibodies in the bone marrow. These antibodies cannot be broken down, and, as a result, they enter the bloodstream and are eventually deposited in other tissues in the form of amyloid proteins.

In contrast to primary amyloidosis, secondary amyloidosis occurs in association with a chronic disease such as tuberculosis, syphilis, rheumatoid arthritis, leprosy, or Hodgkin disease. Secondary amyloidosis often affects the kidneys, liver, and spleen. A particular form of amyloidosis characterized by the deposition of amyloid in the brain is associated with Alzheimer disease.

Hereditary amyloidosis arises when a genetic mutation that causes the formation of amyloid proteins is inherited. There are multiple forms of hereditary amyloidosis. One of the most common forms is known as familial amyloid polyneuropathy (FAP), which is caused by mutations in a gene designated *TTR* (transthyretin). Transthyretin protein, produced by the *TTR* gene, normally circulates in the blood and plays an important role in the transport and tissue delivery of thyroid hormone and retinol. FAP primarily affects the nervous system, resulting in abnormal nerve sensation, pain, and limb weakness. In some cases, amyloid deposits may occur in the heart or kidneys.

Amyloidosis is diagnosed through the detection of amyloid proteins in the blood or urine, as well as through tissue biopsy and imaging studies to locate amyloid deposits within organs. Treatment is directed toward reducing symptoms. Agents commonly prescribed for primary amyloidosis include anti-inflammatory drugs, such as prednisone and colchicine, and some patients may be treated with the chemotherapeutic agent melphalan. In localized forms of the disease, treatment may involve surgical removal of amyloidic masses. In secondary amyloidosis, treatment is aimed at controlling organ damage inflicted by underlying disease. Patients with advanced amyloidosis may require dialysis or liver, heart, or kidney transplant.

Necrotizing Vasculitides

The disorders included in this category are characterized by inflammation of segments of blood vessels, chiefly small and medium-sized arteries. Clinical manifestations depend upon the site and severity of arterial involvement.

No single cause or disease mechanism has been identified for necrotizing vasculitides. In some cases the lesions are similar to those encountered in human serum sickness and in animals given large amounts of foreign protein, in which conditions there is convincing evidence to link the group of disorders to the deposition of immune (antigen-antibody) complexes in the walls of small blood vessels. An antigen (Australia antigen) associated with viral hepatitis (liver inflammation) has been found in the serum of several persons with polyarteritis nodosa, raising the possibility that some cases of polyarteritis may result from the deposition in blood vessels of immune complexes of viral antigen and antibody.

In polyarteritis nodosa, inflammation and necrosis of small and medium-sized arteries lead to local dilation and the formation of small aneurysms. The kidneys are the most frequently involved organs, and the disease is often first manifested by hypertension or other evidence of nephritis (kidney inflammation). Hypersensitivity angiitis tends to involve smaller blood vessels than those affected in polyarteritis nodosa. Frequently, the affected person seems to have experienced hypersensitivity to various medications, particularly penicillin, sulfonamides, and iodides.

Wegener granulomatosis is a disorder marked by the combination of granulomatous lesions of the upper air passages and lower respiratory tract; destructive inflammation of blood vessels, both arteries and veins, especially in the lungs; and localized kidney disease. Treatment includes a combination of immunosuppressive medications, which reduce inflammation and inhibit abnormal cell growth.

Takayasu arteritis, with variants called pulseless disease, branchial arteritis, and giant-cell arteritis of the aorta, involves principally the thoracic aorta (chest portion) and the adjacent segments of its large branches. Symptoms, including diminished or absent pulses in the arms, are related to narrowing and obstruction of these vessels. Takayasu arteritis is most common in young Asian women. The diagnosis and extent of vascular involvement can be established by means of angiography (X-ray observation of the blood vessels). Corticosteroids administered early during the course of the disorder may have a beneficial effect, accompanied on occasion by return of pulses. Anticoagulants may prevent thrombosis (formation of blood clots).

Giant-cell or temporal arteritis occurs chiefly in older people and is manifested by severe temporal or occipital headaches (in the temples or at the back of the head), mental disturbances, visual difficulties, fever, anemia, aching pains and weakness in the muscles of the shoulder and pelvic girdles (polymyalgia rheumatica), and—in a minority of cases—tenderness and nodularity of the temporal artery. This vessel is the site of an inflammation that is characterized by the presence of numerous giant cells. Treatment with small doses of corticosteroids usually leads to relief of symptoms.

Polychondritis and Relapsing Polychondritis

Polychondritis is a chronic disease characterized by inflammation and destruction of the cartilage of various tissues of the body. The cause of polychondritis is unknown, but the disease may be the result of an abnormal immune response. Symptoms include pain, redness, and swelling of the affected cartilage. Polychondritis begins in middle age and most often affects the external ear, nose, and joints. Involvement of the trachea may obstruct breathing or lead to pneumonia. Polychondritis also may affect the inner ear and cause deafness, or it may cause inflammation of the eyes. Corticosteroid medications are administered to moderate the symptoms of the disease, but the effects on the cartilage cannot be reversed.

Relapsing polychondritis is a rare inflammatory disease that primarily affects cartilage. It begins usually in the fourth or fifth decade and is marked by recurrent periods of inflammation of the cartilage of various tissues of the body, lasting several weeks to months. The external ear and nose are affected most frequently and are eventually disfigured ("cauliflower ear") in a high percentage of cases. Eye inflammation also may occur. Involvement of joint cartilages produces pain and swelling of the joints, and the destruction of these cartilages results in a degenerative joint disease that may be disabling. Involvement of the trachea (windpipe) may lead to respiratory obstruction or recurrent pneumonia. The acute manifestations of the disease can usually be suppressed with corticosteroid therapy, but the changes in the cartilage are permanent.

Rheumatoid Arthritis

Rheumatoid arthritis is a chronic, frequently progressive disease in which inflammatory changes occur throughout the connective tissues of the body. Inflammation and thickening of the synovial membranes (the sacs holding the fluid that lubricates the joints) cause irreversible damage to the joint capsule and the articular (joint) cartilage as these structures are replaced by scarlike tissue called pannus. Rheumatoid arthritis is about three times as common in women as in men and afflicts about 1 percent of the adult population in the developed nations. It is much less common than osteoarthritis, which is associated with aging. It primarily affects the middle-aged. (Children are affected by a similar disorder called juvenile rheumatoid arthritis.)

Rheumatoid arthritis usually first attacks joints of the hands and feet symmetrically before progressing to the wrists, knees, or shoulders. The onset of the disorder is gradual. Pain and stiffness in one or more small joints are usually followed by swelling and heat and are accompanied by muscle pain that may become worse, persist for weeks or months, or subside. Joint pain is not always proportionate to the amount of swelling and warmth generated. Fatigue, muscle weakness, and weight loss are common symptoms. Often, before prominent signs appear, the affected person may complain of coldness of hands and feet, numbness, and tingling, all of which suggest compression of the vasomotor nerve.

Active inflammation is first seen in the synovial membranes of the joints, which become red and swollen. Later, a layer of roughened granulation tissue, or pannus, protrudes over the surface of the cartilage. Under the pannus the cartilage is eroded and destroyed. The joints become fixed in place (ankylosed) by thick and hardened pannus, which also may cause displacement and deformity of the joints. The skin, bones, and muscles adjacent to the joints atrophy from disuse and destruction. Painful nodules over bony prominences may persist or regress. Complex collections of cells surrounded by lymphocytes in the connective tissue of muscle and nerve bundles cause pressure and pain; the nodular lesions may invade the connective tissue of the blood vessel walls.

Most persons with rheumatoid arthritis have characteristic autoantibodies in their blood, one of the pieces of evidence implicating an autoimmune mechanism in the disease process. (An autoimmune reaction is an immune reaction against the body's own tissues, and an autoantibody is an antibody that attacks components of the body rather than invading microorganisms.) These autoantibodies are collectively called rheumatoid factor. It is not known what causes the autoimmune reaction, but there is evidence that persons afflicted with the disease have a genetic susceptibility to an environmental agent such as a virus. Once activated by such an agent, a series of immune system reactions causes inflammation.

The most useful medications in relieving the pain and disability of rheumatoid arthritis are aspirin and ibuprofen, which have anti-inflammatory properties. If large doses of these are not sufficient, small doses of corticosteroids such as prednisone may be used. Disease-modifying antirheumatic drugs (DMARDs) also may be prescribed to slow the course of the disease. Physical therapy is helpful in relieving pain and swelling in the affected joints, with an emphasis on the application of heat to the joints followed by exercises that extend the range of motion.

Rest is important, in association with maintaining a good posture to prevent deformity. In cases of severe pain or disability, surgery is used to replace destroyed hip, knee, or finger joints with artificial substitutes. Orthopedic appliances are frequently used to correct or prevent gross deformity and malfunction. The outcome of rheumatoid arthritis is unpredictable, with afflicted individuals either recovering completely or progressing to crippling disease.

Rheumatic Fever

Rheumatic fever is a rare inflammatory disease that is a complication of untreated infection by streptococcus A bacteria. It predominantly affects children between the ages of 5 and 15. Although its name is based upon involvement of the joints, rheumatic fever poses the greatest danger to the heart. The prevalence of rheumatic fever is as high as 3 percent in cases in which streptococcal infection is associated with sore throat and pharyngeal exudate (oozing from the throat surfaces). Persons who have had rheumatic fever are more susceptible to recurrences than the general population is to an initial attack.

Rheumatic fever may be gradual and unnoticed in onset, or it may develop rapidly. Typically, clinical evidence of the disease appears after a symptom-free latent interval of a few days to several weeks after the inciting streptococcal infection. The major indications of its presence in children include inflammation of the heart (especially the valves, manifested by heart murmurs), swollen joints, chorea (a nervous disorder involving unceasing involuntary movements), subcutaneous nodules, and skin rashes, the most characteristic of which is erythema marginatum (reddening of the skin in disk-shaped areas with elevated edges). Fever is common but not invariably present. Symptoms in adults are usually confined to the heart, the joints, or both. Antibiotics, especially penicillin or erythromycin, are employed during the attack to eradicate the streptococci, whereas aspirin, analgesics, and anti-inflammatory medications are used to treat the acute symptoms. Unless there is damage to heart valves, recovery usually is complete. Scarring and deformity of the valves may lead to their narrowing or failure to close properly, and this may eventually lead to the development of heart failure. The prophylactic use of antibiotics (chiefly penicillin) has led to a dramatic reduction in the frequency of streptococcal infections and resultant recurrences of rheumatic fever.

Several antibodies against streptococcus develop in response to infection. These are directed against various constituents of the microorganism or its products. The mechanisms whereby streptococcal infection initiates the process of rheumatic fever appear to be immunological in nature and to be based in large measure on antigenic reactions between a protein constituent of the streptococcal cell walls and human heart tissue and between other fractions of the streptococcus and a component of joint cartilage. Immunoglobulins produced in response to these bacterial antigens may act as autoantibodies and be responsible for the inflammation of the heart and joints.

Scleroderma

Scleroderma is a chronic disease of the skin that also can affect the blood vessels and various internal organs. Scleroderma is characterized by excessive deposition of collagen—the principal supportive protein of the connective tissues—in affected areas. There are two main types of scleroderma: a systemic form called progressive systemic scleroderma, which can be life-threatening, and a localized form, which is usually not as serious.

The term *scleroderma*, which means "hard skin," indicates the hardening and thickening of the skin that is the most common feature of the disease. Scleroderma strikes women more often than men and may begin at any age, although symptoms commonly appear in persons between ages 25 and 50. In cases of localized scleroderma, isolated patches of hardened skin are often the only sign of the disease. Occasionally muscles and bone are involved, but no internal organs are affected. In cases of progressive systemic scleroderma, however, many parts of the body may be involved, including the skin, blood vessels, kidneys, lungs, heart, and gastrointestinal tract. The severity of systemic scleroderma depends on which organs are affected and to what degree they become damaged. Those with

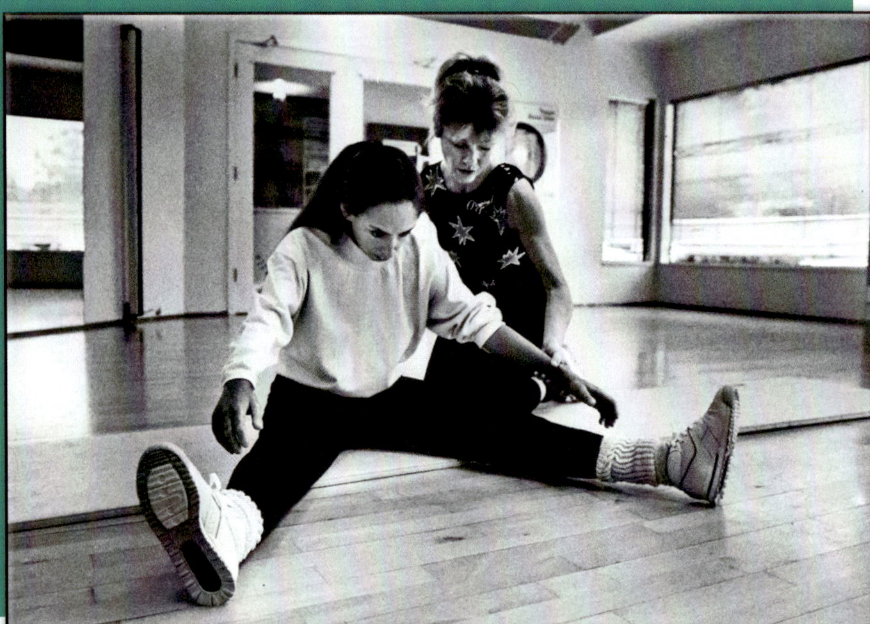

An aerobics instructor helps a scleroderma patient stretch. The hardening of skin and connective tissue that is symptomatic of this condition can make movement difficult. Stretching helps maintain suppleness. John Storey/Time & Life Pictures/Getty Images

localized scleroderma do not usually develop systemic scleroderma.

The onset of progressive systemic scleroderma usually is marked by hands and feet changing colour from pale to blue to red in response to cold, a manifestation called Raynaud phenomenon that is caused by abnormal blood flow. As the disease progresses, the facial skin often tightens into a shiny mask. Swelling may occur, along with skin discoloration, numbness, and a tingling feeling. The course of the disease is variable and unpredictable. Sometimes years intervene between the early manifestations and the more serious signs of systemic involvement, which may include difficulty in breathing or swallowing, gastrointestinal disorders, kidney malfunction, and inflammation of the heart lining, heart muscle, or sac enclosing the heart. If heart, lung, or kidney dysfunction occurs early in the course of the disease, the prognosis is poor.

There is a milder variant of progressive systemic scleroderma, called CREST syndrome. The acronym is derived from the first letters of the five main features of the disease:

- *C*alcinosis cutis, calcium deposits in the skin
- *R*aynaud phenomenon
- *E*sophageal dysfunction
- *S*clerodactyly, tightening of the skin on the fingers and toes
- *T*elangiectasia, red spots on the face, lips, forearms, and hands

The signs and symptoms of scleroderma arise because the tissue of the targeted organ is inflamed and irritated and eventually becomes scarred and loses normal elasticity. These changes occur as a result of an increase in the deposition of collagen in the targeted areas. Collagen overproduction is thought to result from an autoimmune reaction—i.e., a malfunctioning of the immune system that causes the body to attack its own components. The stimulus that results in this derangement of the immune system is not known.

No cure has been found for scleroderma, but treatments are available that help alleviate its symptoms. For example, corticosteroids help reduce inflammation, and immunosuppressants and other drugs help soften the skin. Heat, massage, and physical therapy are often of value, and sometimes a change of climate can bring about improvement.

Sjögren Syndrome

Sjögren syndrome, also called sicca syndrome, is a chronic inflammatory disorder characterized by severe dryness of the eyes and the mouth that results from a diminution in secretion of tears and saliva. Dryness may also involve the nose, pharynx, larynx, and tracheobronchial tree. Approximately half the persons affected also have rheumatoid arthritis or, less commonly, some other connective-tissue disease, such as scleroderma, polymyositis, or systemic lupus erythematosus. The great majority of the persons affected by Sjögren syndrome are women.

Infiltration (gradual assemblage) of lymphocytes and plasma cells leads to enlargement of the parotid or other salivary glands in half the patients. There may also be enlargement of the spleen, diminution in white blood cell numbers, Raynaud phenomenon, vasculitis (inflammation of vessels) with chronic leg ulcers, a disease of the peripheral or trigeminal nerves, chronic (Hashimoto) thyroiditis (inflammation of the thyroid), enlargement of the liver, and inflammation of the pancreas. A number of persons with sicca syndrome of long duration have developed neoplasms of the type called reticulum cell sarcoma, or primary macroglobulinemia (the presence in the blood of globulins of high molecular weight).

Treatment toward relief of symptoms includes the administration of artificial tears to lessen ocular dryness. Corticosteroids or immunosuppressive drugs have been employed with some success for the more serious manifestations.

SYSTEMIC LUPUS ERYTHEMATOSUS

Systemic lupus erythematosus (SLE) is a chronic inflammatory disease of unknown cause that affects, either singularly or in combination, the skin, joints, kidneys, nervous system, and membranes lining body cavities and often other organs as well. The disease has a tendency toward remissions and exacerbations and a multitude of immunologic abnormalities, including antibodies that react with components of cell nuclei, as well as antibodies directed against circulating proteins, blood cells, and solid organs. The disease may develop at any period of life but appears with highest frequency during the second to fourth decades. Most affected persons are women, and the disorder is three times more common in black women than in white women. Systemic lupus erythematosus exists in many forms, from the very mild to severe and rapidly fatal. The annual incidence of the disease has been estimated to be at least three to six cases per 100,000 population.

The identification of systemic lupus erythematosus is based primarily on certain clinical findings, the most specific and frequent of which include: (1) facial erythema (reddening), which often takes the form of a butterfly-shaped rash over the bridge of the nose and the cheeks and which occurs in only a minority of adults with the disease, (2) discoid lupus, an erythematous raised patchy

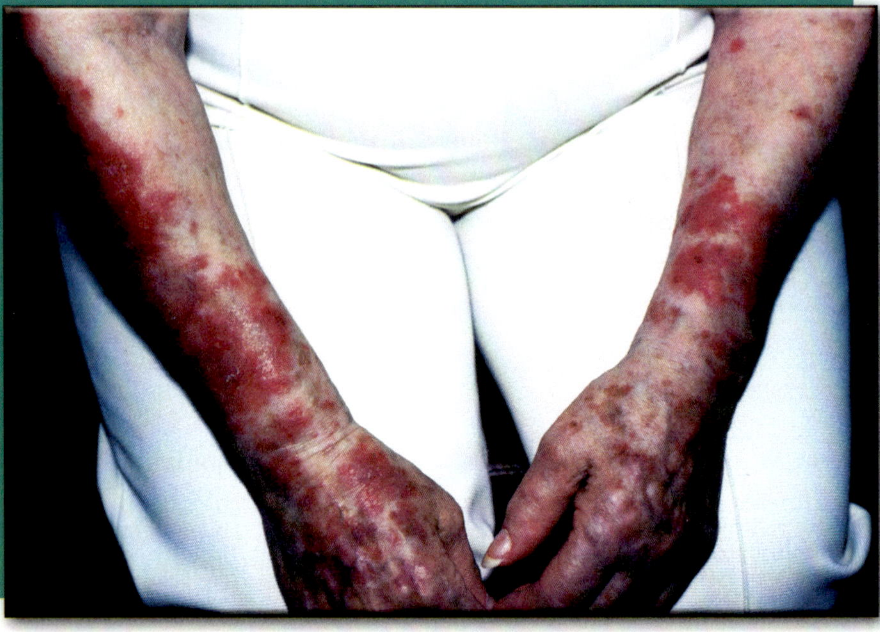

In addition to the telltale butterfly-shaped rash on their faces, patients with lupus may develop severe skin rashes elsewhere on the body. CMSP/ Collection Mix: Subjects/Getty Images

eruption that heals with scarring and atrophy of the skin and may be found anywhere on the body, (3) Raynaud syndrome, (4) photosensitivity, manifested by unusual skin reaction after exposure to sunlight, (5) nondeforming arthritis, (6) inflammation of the kidneys (glomerulonephritis), (7) inflammation of the chest lining (pleurisy) or of the membranous sac enclosing the heart (pericarditis), or both, and (8) central nervous system involvement, in the form of psychosis or convulsions. In addition to specific organ involvement, affected persons also have constitutional symptoms—including fever, weakness, fatigability, and weight loss—that are often the first manifestation of illness.

Some degree of anemia is found in most persons with the disease, often the result of an increased rate of red cell destruction attributable to antibodies that coat the cell and damage its membrane. Low white blood cell counts (leukopenia) and platelet counts (thrombocytopenia) are also characteristic; these too can often be traced to the presence of specific autoantibodies. Abnormal bleeding may result from thrombocytopenia or from an antibody that combines with and inactivates certain plasma proteins (clotting factors) involved in blood coagulation. Rheumatoid factor occurs in about 25 percent of cases. Most important from the standpoint of diagnosis are the antibodies that combine with various components of cell nuclei. One or more of these antinuclear antibodies are present in virtually all persons with active disease. The first of these antibodies to be recognized was the lupus erythematosus cell factor, discovery of which permitted detection of previously obscure and unrecognized forms of systemic lupus erythematosus.

The compound thus formed is avidly ingested by certain phagocytic (particle-engulfing) white blood cells called neutrophilic leukocytes, which, distended by the compound of antibody and of lymphocyte-nucleus component, are the characteristic lupus erythematosus cells. Two antibodies fairly characteristic of lupus erythematosus react specifically with deoxyribonucleic acid (DNA) and double-stranded ribonucleic acid (RNA) of cell nuclei. The presence of these two antibodies is associated with an active disease, in particular with inflammation of the kidney and with skin and brain lesions. Evidence strongly suggests the possibility that one or more viruses may be the ultimate source of the antigenic stimulation responsible for the development of these autoantibodies.

The treatment of systemic lupus erythematosus aims to reduce or control inflammation and to limit damage to vital organs. Salicylates (aspirin) are used to relieve pain, particularly when joints are involved, and to reduce fever.

In most cases, it is necessary to employ corticosteroid hormones or NSAIDs (nonsteroidal anti-inflammatory drugs) to reduce inflammation in acute crises of the disease. Certain antimalarial medications, such as chloroquine and hydroxychloroquine, have been found to exert an anti-inflammatory effect on skin and joint lesions and are widely used for the treatment of milder forms of the disease. Immunosuppressive medications are prescribed for patients whose kidneys or central nervous systems are affected by the disease.

The course of systemic lupus erythematosus is highly variable. Acute episodes occur, but more commonly the disease gives rise to a subacute or chronic illness that smolders for many months or years, subject to spontaneous remissions and exacerbations. There may be long intervals (up to 20 years or more) in which the affected person is entirely free of symptoms, with little or no evidence of the disease aside from serologic abnormalities, which tend to persist indefinitely. In most cases the prospects of survival are determined by the degree of kidney involvement and its responsiveness to treatment with corticosteroids and other measures. Persons with severe and persistent thrombocytopenia (deficiency of blood platelets) and hemolytic anemia or with central nervous system disease fare poorly compared with those whose illness mainly involves the joints.

There are a number of medications that have been found to be responsible for the induction of a lupuslike disease. Typically, this disease is manifested by the appearance of fever, joint pain, pleurisy, deficiency of white blood cells, and the development of various antinuclear antibodies (antibodies that interact with cell nuclei). The clinical features thus closely resemble those of lupus, with the exception that evidence of kidney involvement is notably rare, and the symptoms generally disappear upon discontinuation of the offending drug. Medications that have had this effect include hydralazine, procainamide, various anticonvulsants, isoniazid, penicillin, and penicillamine. In one study, these or other drugs were found to account for 3 to 12 percent of all the cases identified as lupus. Only a small proportion of persons who receive these drugs present evidence of a lupuslike disease.

Thrombotic Thrombocytopenic Purpura

Thrombotic thrombocytopenic purpura is a rare disorder that is included with the connective tissue diseases chiefly because of certain clinical similarities to systemic lupus erythematosus. The main features of this disorder, which usually appears suddenly in young women, include thrombocytopenic purpura (presence in the skin of red spots from the escape of blood into the tissues as a result of scarcity of blood platelets), hemolytic anemia (anemia resulting from destruction of red blood cells), changing neurological manifestations, fever, and kidney failure. There is widespread blockage of small blood vessels—arterioles, venules, and capillaries—by material consisting principally of fibrin, the principal constituent of blood clots. The heart, kidneys, and brain are particularly affected. Treatment includes plasmapheresis, a procedure that removes antigen-antibody complexes from the blood. Surgical removal of the spleen may be necessary if affected individuals do not respond to this treatment or have frequent recurrences of the disease.

OTHER DISORDERS INVOLVING CONNECTIVE TISSUES

There exists a variety of disorders of connective tissue that involve inflammation but that are not necessarily associated with a disorder of autoimmunity. Such disorders typically involve physical damage to the primary connective tissue structures (e.g., tendons, ligaments, collagen, and bone), which produces symptoms of pain and inflammation. Common disorders of this nature include carpal tunnel syndrome, herniation of the cartilage disks in the vertebral column, and tendinitis. Although some level of autoimmune response has been implicated in polychondritis (the inflammation and subsequent deterioration of cartilage), because the condition can involve extensive damage to primary connective tissues, it is considered here.

Carpal Tunnel Syndrome

Carpal tunnel syndrome (CTS) is a condition of numbness, tingling, or pain in the wrist that is caused by repetitive flexing or stressing of the fingers or wrist over a long period of time. Possibly the most common repetitive stress injury in the workplace, CTS is frequently associated with the modern office, where the computer has transformed the nature of the work people do with their hands and arms.

CTS is caused by pressure on the median nerve, a soft structure filled with fibres that carry nerve impulses back and forth between the hand and the spinal cord via the wrist joint. The wrist joint is formed by two rows of bones called the carpal bones (from Greek *karpos*, "wrist"). The carpal tunnel is a small passage almost completely surrounded by the carpal bones. On the inner, or palm, side of the wrist, the tunnel is enclosed by a tight band of fibrous tissue called the transverse carpal ligament. Through the tunnel run the median nerve, several blood vessels, and nine finger flexor tendons. The tendons are rodlike structures that transmit forces from muscles in the forearm to the fingers and enable the fingers to close, as when making a fist.

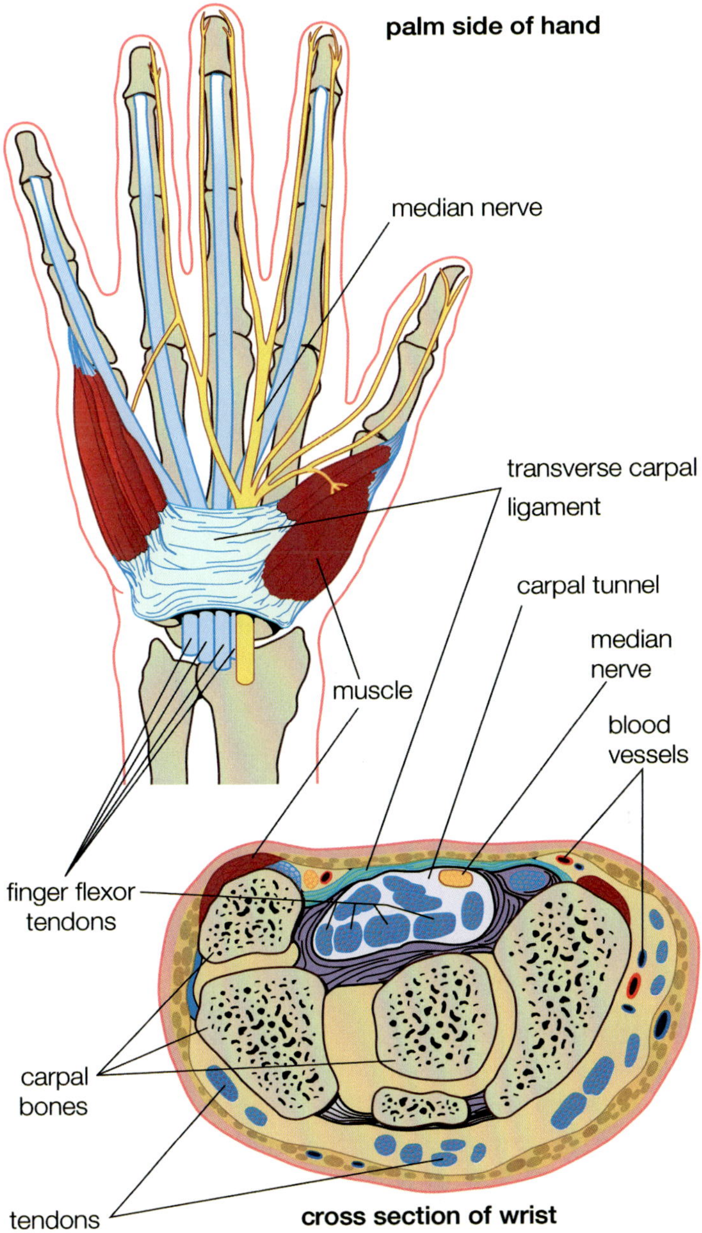

The structures of the wrist associated with carpal tunnel syndrome. Encyclopædia Britannica, Inc.

During movements of the fingers and wrist, the finger flexor tendons rub against the walls of the carpal tunnel and the median nerve itself. Although the tendons are lubricated by a special tendon lining and by synovial fluid, certain repetitive movements, especially in combination with forceful gripping, may cause swelling of the tendons or the sheaths surrounding them. Because there is little room for expansion within the tight confinement of the carpal tunnel, the result of swelling is that the softest tissues—the median nerve and blood vessels—become compressed or pinched. This pressure causes the numbness, tingling, and pain in the wrist and hand that are the primary symptoms of CTS. If pressure on the median nerve increases, affected individuals may experience a temporary loss of control of some of the hand muscles and difficulties in picking up or holding objects. They may also be awakened at night by pain in the hand.

CTS can occur in individuals who do repeated, forceful gripping and grasping hand motions—as in the use of clippers, pliers, or power drills—as a result of stress over the base of the palm, where the median nerve is protected only by the 3-mm- (0.1-inch-) thick transverse carpal ligament. Leaning the wrists on a desk or table while operating a computer can also place excessive pressure on the median nerve and may result in inflammation of the tendons and tissues surrounding the nerve. However, not all cases of CTS are work-related. Illnesses that cause tissue inflammation—for example, arthritis, gout, hypothyroidism, or diabetes mellitus—may affect the median nerve within the carpal tunnel. Swelling and bleeding associated with a fracture of the wrist may also put undue pressure on the nerve.

For cases of CTS caused by non-work-related problems, treatment is aimed at the underlying condition. If a case is caused by repetitive stress, then avoiding or reducing the activity responsible for the syndrome will often rapidly alleviate the symptoms. Frequent resting of the hand and recourse to stretching exercises for the hands, elbows, shoulders, and neck muscles will decrease symptoms over a period of time. The wearing of a brace or splint will support the wrist, relieve overworked wrist structures, and help to prevent reinjury of healing tissues. The taking of nonsteroidal anti-inflammatory medications such as aspirin or ibuprofen will frequently reduce swelling of the tendon sheaths. More-serious cases can be relieved immediately by the injection of prescription steroidal drugs. Surgery is also sometimes necessary to correct the condition. Whether done as a traditional open incision or as less-invasive endoscopy, the surgery aims to relieve pressure within the carpal tunnel by cutting the transverse carpal ligament. Surgery can be performed on an outpatient basis, but healing and recovery can take weeks or months.

Herniated Disk

A herniated disk (also known as a protruded, or slipped, disk) is a displacement of part of the rubbery centre, or nucleus, of a cartilaginous disk from between the vertebrae so that it presses against the spinal cord. Pain occurs in the arms if the protrusion occurs at the level of the neck (between the fifth and sixth or sixth and seventh cervical vertebrae) or in the lower back and legs if the protrusion occurs low in the backbone (usually between the fourth and fifth lumbar vertebrae or between the fifth lumbar and first sacral vertebrae). Treatment, depending on the severity of the condition, may include bed rest, analgesic medication (e.g., aspirin), traction, orthopedic support, and physical therapy or surgical removal of the protruded portion of the disk and fusion of the spinal vertebrae at the point affected.

Polychondritis

Polychondritis is a chronic disease characterized by inflammation and destruction of the cartilage of various tissues of the body. The cause of polychondritis is unknown, but the disease may be the result of an abnormal immune response. Symptoms include pain, redness, and swelling of the affected cartilage. Polychondritis begins in middle age and most often affects the external ear, nose, and joints. Involvement of the trachea may obstruct breathing or lead to pneumonia. Polychondritis also may affect the inner ear and cause deafness, or it may cause inflammation of the eyes. Corticosteroid medications are administered to moderate the symptoms of the disease, but the effects on the cartilage cannot be reversed.

Tendinitis

Tendinitis (also spelled tendonitis) is an inflammation of the sheaths of the tendons. These sheaths are composed of thin, filmy tissue that permits the sliding motion of tendons within them. The cause of inflammation is irritation of the sheaths by prolonged or abnormal use of the tendons. Less often it may follow invasion of the tendon sheaths by bacteria with subsequent infection. It is in many instances an occupational hazard (wrist tendons in the typist, tendons about the shoulder in baseball pitchers, or tendons about the elbow in pneumatic drill operators).

Inflammation in the sheath of the tendon produces swelling, redness, and pain along the course of the involved tendon, and motion of the tendon produces severe pain. Swelling of the sheath narrows the space through which the tendon may slide, causing stiffness in the involved area. A grating sensation may be felt as the tendon moves.

Treatment of the condition involves placing the involved tendon and its sheath at complete rest by means of splints, a cast, or bandages. With rest the inflammation subsides, and motion may gradually be resumed. Administration of anti-inflammatory medications or local injections of corticosteroids may hasten the abatement of the inflammation. Recurrences following improvement are not uncommon. Repeated episodes of tendinitis may produce permanent thickening of the sheath, which limits motion of the tendon within it. Surgery may be necessary in severe cases of tendinitis.

CHAPTER 8

CANCERS AND HEREDITARY DISORDERS OF THE SKIN AND CONNECTIVE TISSUE

Cancers of the skin and connective tissue, which may be hereditary or acquired, can cause extensive damage to not only localized areas of these tissues but surrounding or even distant tissues as well. Perhaps the best known and most common of these diseases is skin cancer.

Hereditary disorders of skin and connective tissue are a heterogeneous group. Many of these are single-gene disorders, meaning that they arise from defects in a single gene that affect one or another of the primary elements of the connective tissues. Many of these defects cause skeletal and joint abnormalities that may interfere seriously with normal growth and development.

COMMON CANCERS OF SKIN AND CONNECTIVE TISSUE

Cancers of the skin and connective tissue arise from abnormalities in the cells that form these tissues. Thus, the different types of cancers of these tissues are distinguished by the types of cells involved. Melanoma, for example, is a cancer of the pigment-producing melanocytes, and sarcoma is a cancer of cells of the mesoderm, hence producing disease in connective tissue. Skin cancers and major forms of sarcomas are discussed in the following sections.

Melanoma

Melanoma is a spreading and frequently recurring cancer of the melanocytes, which produce the protective skin-darkening pigment melanin. According to data published in 2009 by the World Health Organization, an estimated 132,000 new melanoma cases are diagnosed worldwide each year. In the United States melanoma represents nearly 5 percent of all cases of cancer.

Melanoma is a deadly disease. It is responsible for nearly three-quarters of all skin cancer deaths and is increasing in frequency. Unlike other skin growths, melanoma is always malignant.

Causes and Symptoms

People vary in their susceptibility to melanoma. Whites are 20 times more likely to develop melanoma than are blacks. People who have fair skin or who freckle easily are particularly susceptible. Individuals with a large number of moles or with several very large moles are also at increased risk. Similar to all cancers, melanoma is caused by changes in DNA that alter a cell's ability to control its growth. The most common cause of DNA damage in melanocytes is ultraviolet radiation from sunlight. In some cases DNA mutations that cause melanoma or that increase the risk of the cancer can be inherited.

Between 50 and 70 percent of melanomas are caused by spontaneous mutations in a gene known as *BRAF*, which produces a protein called B-raf. B-raf is a kinase—a type of enzyme specializing in the transmission of intracellular signals from cell surface receptors to proteins that communicate with the cell nucleus. B-raf plays a central role in the carefully regulated transmission of cellular signals that result in the stimulation of cell differentiation and in the suppression of programmed cell death (apoptosis). However, activating mutations in the *BRAF* gene result in the production of a constantly active, unregulated B-raf kinase. This mutant enzyme is programmed to transmit signals continuously, regardless of whether or not it is instructed to do so by cell surface receptors. This aberrant activity results in uncontrolled cell proliferation, thereby initiating the generation of cancer cells that give rise to melanoma. Mutations in *BRAF* appear to be acquired as a result of overexposure to ultraviolet radiation.

Other genetic variants have been linked to melanoma. A number of mutations in a gene called *MCR1* occur in association with mutations in *BRAF*. *MCR1* mutations also are sometimes involved in melanomas that develop

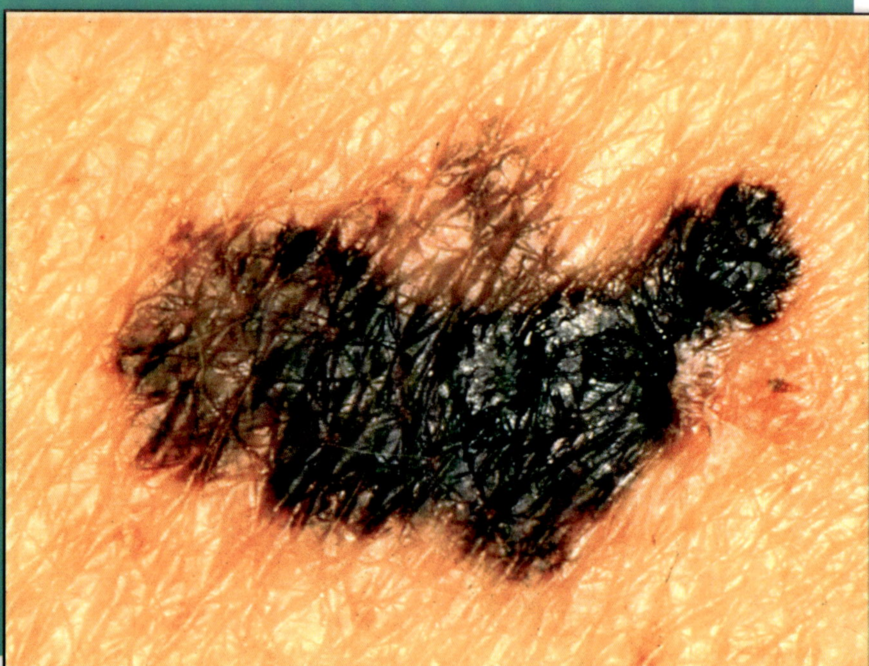

A pathology image of melanoma. The deadliest form of skin cancer, melanoma may present as an irregularly shaped/coloured mole. Skin Cancer Foundation

independent of exposure to ultraviolet light. Mutations in a tumour suppressor gene known as *CDKN2A*, which produces a kinase involved in regulating the cell cycle and cell division, have been associated with cutaneous malignant melanoma, an inherited form of the disease.

The earliest symptoms of melanoma are often visual. Large or abnormally coloured moles on the surface of the skin are early indicators. Melanoma can be detected in its early stages by regular self-assessment of moles, using the ABCD system. ABCD stands for asymmetry, border, colour, and diameter. Moles that are asymmetrical, have irregular borders (edges) or colour, or are greater than 5–6 mm (about ¼ inch) in diameter are suspect. Any mole that changes in size, shape, or colour should be examined by a physician immediately.

Diagnosis and Treatment

Following the identification of a potential melanoma, diagnosis is made by skin biopsy. A sample of the skin is examined under a microscope for signs of cancer growth and for measurement of the thickness of the growth. If melanoma is diagnosed, several treatment options are available. The most widely used treatments include surgery, chemotherapy, and radiation therapy. In addition, some patients receive biological therapy, in which agents designed to mimic substances naturally occurring in the body are used to fight cancer or to counter side effects of certain anticancer drugs.

The treatment approach to melanoma is based on the severity or stage of the disease. Stage 0 through stage II melanomas are confined to the skin, and most of these can be cured by excision of the tumour, especially if caught early. Some patients with stage II melanoma may undergo selective sentinel lymphadenectomy, which entails the removal of lymph nodes most likely to be the first affected by metastasizing (spreading) cancer cells. Stage II patients also may be treated with biological agents, such as interferon or bevacizumab (Avastin; a monoclonal antibody), following surgery. Stage III melanoma has spread to nearby lymph nodes, and surgical removal of the cancerous nodes is required. This may be followed by biological therapy or chemotherapy. Stage IV melanoma has spread beyond the regional lymph nodes to other tissues in the body and is extremely serious. No cure for stage IV melanoma is available, but disease progression may be delayed by surgery and by the administration of chemotherapy, biological therapy, or radiation therapy. Unfortunately, the survival rate for stage IV melanoma is extremely low.

Prevention

The risk of melanoma is greatly reduced by avoiding exposure to ultraviolet light. Exposure can be reduced by staying out of direct sunlight during periods of peak intensity (11:00 AM to 3:00 PM), protecting the skin with clothing, or using a sunscreen with an SPF rating of 15 or higher. Children should be particularly careful to avoid sunburns, as an increased risk of developing melanoma has been linked to severe sunburns during childhood. Ultraviolet-sensitive devices that warn of potential overexposure to sunlight in order to prevent sunburn are being developed. These devices, which could be worn around the wrist, indicate the increasing risk of sunburn by using simple colour changes that are induced by ultraviolet rays.

Nonmelanoma Skin Cancer

Nonmelanoma skin cancers are cancers of surface tissues (carcinomas). There are two forms of nonmelanoma, both of which can usually be cured with minor surgery. Squamous cell carcinomas develop from a layer of flat cells close to the skin's surface and account for about one-fourth of nonmelanoma cases. Basal cell carcinomas account for roughly three-fourths of cases, and recurrence of this cancer is common. Basal cell carcinoma begins in a layer of cells underlying the squamous cells. The squamous and basal cell layers are both located in the epidermis.

Causes and Symptoms

Most cases of nonmelanoma skin cancer are caused by damage to DNA resulting from exposure to ultraviolet radiation of the sun. People with light complexions have a higher rate of skin cancer than those with dark skin, and males are more likely to develop skin cancer than females. Exposure to substances such as arsenic, coal, and tar has been linked to skin cancer, as has infection with human papillomavirus (HPV), particularly those infections causing genital warts. Other factors that increase skin cancer rates are chronic inflammatory skin diseases, long-term treatment for psoriasis, previous radiation treatment, and immune suppression. The rare congenital disorders xeroderma pigmentosum and basal cell nevus are also associated with increased risk.

The predominant symptom of nonmelanoma skin cancer is an unusual growth, mole, or other abnormal appearance on the skin. Abnormalities may be raised or flat and may be red, pink, black, blue, brown, or flesh-coloured. Moles or growths that are new, that grow or change shape rapidly, or that will not heal are particular signs of skin cancer and should be examined by a dermatologist.

Diagnosis and Prognosis

If cancer is suspected, a diagnosis is made following a skin biopsy. Depending on the severity of the skin lesion, a biopsy can be conducted by scraping surface cells, by using a narrow punch to extract a larger tissue sample, or by excising a section of skin and surrounding tissue with a scalpel.

Once nonmelanoma skin cancer has been diagnosed, its stage is determined to indicate how far the cancer has progressed. Stage 0 skin cancer is also called squamous cell carcinoma in situ, or Bowen disease, and is confined to the epidermis. Stage I cancers are 2 cm (approximately ¾ inch) or less in size; stage II, more than 2 cm. Neither has spread beyond the skin. Stage III cancers have spread to deeper layers of the skin, underlying tissues, or nearby lymph nodes. Stage IV cancers have spread to other parts of the body such as the muscles, bones, lungs, nerves, or brain.

Very few cases of nonmelanoma spread to other tissues before they are detected and removed. Basal cell carcinomas rarely spread to surrounding tissues, and five-year survival rates approach 100 percent when these cancers are detected early, as most are. A small percentage of basal cell carcinomas spread to nearby lymph nodes and surrounding tissues; the five-year survival rate in these cases is very low. Squamous cell carcinomas also have an extremely high five-year survival rate when detected early, but the rate drops considerably if the cancer has spread.

Treatment

If diagnosed early, nonmelanoma skin cancers can be cured with minor surgery to remove the affected tissue. Removal may be accomplished by a simple surgical excision, by freezing the cells with liquid nitrogen, or by destroying them with a laser. In some superficial cancers the cells may be removed by merely scraping them off; any residual cancer cells are then killed with pulses of electricity. A procedure known as Moh surgery shaves off cells one layer at a time, stopping when microscopic analysis indicates that no cancer remains. In some cases, removal of nearby lymph nodes may also be necessary.

Radiation therapy can be used to cure very small cancers or to delay progression of larger cancers. It is sometimes used in conjunction with surgery to kill any cancer cells left behind. Side effects of radiation treatment may include vomiting, diarrhea, fatigue, or skin irritation resembling a sunburn or suntan.

Chemotherapy is sometimes used to treat skin cancers by directly applying a chemotherapeutic agent to the affected tissue; this reduces side effects, which can resemble those of radiation treatment. In the rare cases when nonmelanoma has spread to distant tissues, systemic chemotherapy may be necessary, although it generally will not cure the cancer.

Prevention

Skin cancer can be prevented by avoiding risk factors, particularly exposure to ultraviolet radiation from the sun. Sunlamps and tanning beds should be avoided, and the skin should be protected with sunscreen or clothing when outdoors. Some medical societies recommend a skin examination by a physician every three years for people between the ages of 20 and 40 and yearly examinations thereafter. Regular self-examinations of the skin are also recommended, and any unusual growth or appearance should be checked by a physician.

Cancers of Connective Tissues

Cancers of connective tissues are often referred to generally as sarcomas. Sarcoma is relatively rare in adults but is one of the more common malignancies among children. It often spreads to other tissues in the body. Sarcomas are generally divided into bone and soft-tissue tumours, the latter being much less common. Because mesenchymal cells form a variety of mature tissues, tumours may have the characteristics of bone (osteosarcoma), cartilage (chondrosarcoma), muscle (myosarcoma), or blood vessels (angiosarcoma). The varieties overlap, and the name given to the sarcoma is taken from that of the most developed tissue contained within the tumour. The most common is osteosarcoma. This malignancy of immature bone (osteoid) was highly lethal before the use of anticancer drugs, which have increased the survival rate to about 90 percent. Specific chromosomal abnormalities are associated with some sarcomas.

Chondrosarcoma is a rare malignant tumour of bone formed from cartilage. Pain is the most common symptom. Primary chondrosarcomas arise from a small collection of cartilage cells. The secondary type develops slowly from a previously benign tumour of cartilage. The tumour may mestastasize to the lungs in some cases. An extremely rare form of chondrosarcoma also may occur as a primary tumour in soft tissues and muscle without involvement of the bone. Middle-aged and elderly persons are most often affected, and the tumours are twice as common in males. Treatment includes surgical removal of the tumour.

Fibrosarcoma is a rare malignant tumour of fibrous tissue most commonly found in middle-age adults and primarily occurring in the thighbone, upper arm bone, or jaw. The tumour also may arise in soft tissues and organs. The mass is detectable by palpation before pain occurs. The tumour may invade surrounding tissues, which makes complete surgical excision difficult. It often recurs, and it may metastasize if the cells are large, have bizarre shapes, and are abundantly replicating. Tumours with cells that have a less unusual appearance have a much better prognosis.

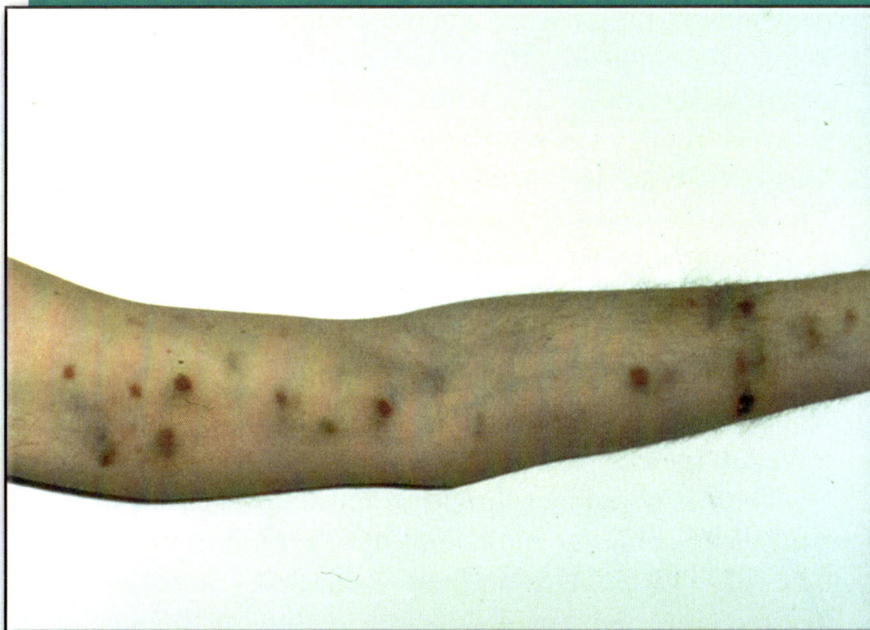

Karposi sarcoma lesions on the arm of an AIDS patient. This form of cancer attacks the tissue beneath the skin's surface or mucus membranes first, and may spread to other organs. National Cancer Institute

Kaposi sarcoma, also called idiopathic multiple pigmented hemorrhagic sarcoma, is a rare and usually lethal cancer of the tissues beneath the surface of the skin or of the mucous membranes. The disease can spread to other organs, including the liver, lungs, and intestinal tract. Kaposi sarcoma is characterized by red-purple or blue-brown lesions of the skin, mucous membranes, and other organs. The skin lesions may be firm or compressible, solitary or clustered. Kaposi sarcoma primarily occurs in people afflicted with acquired immunodeficiency syndrome (AIDS).

Kaposi sarcoma was considered an extremely rare cancer until about 1980, when the disease became increasingly evident in AIDS patients. Kaposi sarcoma, in fact, was the disease that indicated the presence of AIDS in nearly half of the cases reported to the U.S. Centers for Disease Control. Young male homosexuals with AIDS are far more likely to develop the cancer than are other AIDS patients. The breakdown of the immune system and the production of a growth factor by white blood cells infected with HIV (human immunodeficiency virus), the virus that causes AIDS, seem to encourage the sarcoma's occurrence—i.e., it is considered an opportunistic tumour. The development of Kaposi sarcoma is also thought to be linked to infection by the herpes virus HHV-8.

There is no known cure for Kaposi sarcoma, although partial and complete remissions have been accomplished. The AIDS patient is nonetheless subject to a return of the disease. However, the introduction of antiviral therapy for those infected with HIV has reduced the incidence of the sarcoma. The disease is named after Mortiz Kaposi, who first reported it in 1872.

HEREDITARY DISORDERS OF SKIN AND CONNECTIVE TISSUE

There are a number of different hereditary disorders of skin and connective tissue. These conditions may be inherited in one of several ways, including as an autosomal dominant or autosomal recessive trait. Autosomal dominant traits are those in which the inheritance of a single copy of the mutant gene from one parent is sufficient to cause disease. Autosomal recessive traits are those in which the inheritance of two copies of the mutant gene, one from each parent, is required to cause disease. Notable among these disorders are achondroplasia, Ehlers-Danlos syndrome, Marfan syndrome, and osteogenesis imperfecta.

Achondroplasia

Achondroplasia, or chondrodystrophia fetalis, is a genetic disorder characterized by an abnormality in the conversion of cartilage into bone. As a consequence, bones that depend on cartilage models for development, particularly long bones such as the femur and humerus, cannot grow. Achondroplasia is the most common cause of dwarfism. In those afflicted with the disorder, the limbs are very short (fingers reach only to the hips), but the trunk is almost normal in size. The head is enlarged because of some overgrowth of the vault bones following premature closure of sutures at the base of the skull. Other manifestations of achrondoplasia include a bulging forehead, saddle nose, protruding jaw, deeply incurved lower back with prominent buttocks, and a narrow chest; women with the disorder may have narrow pelvises and, subsequently, difficulty in childbirth. Achondroplasia is inherited as an autosomal dominant trait. However, about 80 percent of cases of the disorder result from new genetic mutations rather than from the parental transmission of defective genes. Affected individuals are of normal intelligence and have otherwise normal health.

Alkaptonuria

Alkaptonuria is a rare inherited (autosomal recessive) disorder in which the absence of the liver and kidney enzyme homogentisic acid oxidase results in an abnormal accumulation of homogentisic acid, a normal intermediate in the metabolism of the amino acid tyrosine. Alkaptonuria is rather rare, occurring in one in 200,000 births.

Some homogentisic acid is excreted in the urine, to which, upon alkalinization and oxidation, it imparts a black colour. However, except for a blackening of the urine, this disorder has no clinical manifestations until the affected person is around age 20 or 30, when deposits of ochre pigments begin to appear in various fibrous connective tissues of the body. The pigment, bound to collagen fibres in the deeper layers of joint cartilage and intervertebral disks (the fibrous pads between adjacent bones of the spine), causes these tissues to lose their normal resiliency and become brittle. The erosion of the abnormal cartilage leads to a progressive degenerative disease of the joints, which usually becomes manifest by the fourth decade of life. Usually, the intervertebral disks become thinned and calcified first, and later the knees, shoulders, and hips are affected.

Alkaptonuria is compatible with normal life expectancy. In some cases arteriosclerosis has been described. However, it is not known whether this is a manifestation of the disease or coincidental. No effective treatment is available for the underlying metabolic disorder.

Dupuytren Contracture

Dupuytren contracture is a flexion deformity of the hands caused by thickening of the fascia, or fibrous connective tissue, of the palm. The proliferation of connective tissue causes the tendons of one or more fingers to shorten and tighten, leaving the finger permanently flexed. Disability may be as slight as inability to extend the ring finger completely or as severe as complete curling of the hand into a closed fist. The contracture does not affect neighbouring nerves and other structures. Dupuytren contracture may be inherited or may occur as a symptom of scleroderma or rheumatoid arthritis. In some severe cases, incision and removal of some of the connective tissue may release the contracture.

Ehlers-Danlos Syndrome

Ehlers-Danlos syndrome is manifested particularly by an abnormal skin elasticity and fragility and by loose-jointedness. The skin, peculiarly stretchable even in early childhood, gradually loses its elasticity. Minor injury can cause lacerations that tend to bleed severely and to extend. Scoliosis (lateral curvature of the spine), recurrent dislocations of joints, and hernias of the abdominal wall or the diaphragm (the muscular partition between the chest and the abdomen) are seen as in Marfan syndrome, and there may be blue sclerae (the "whites" of the eye). The underlying defect of the disorder has not been determined, but it is likely that it involves the abnormal organization of collagen bundles. Some researchers have also detected an excess of elastin fibres in the connective tissue of persons with the disease. It is now clear that there are at least 10 distinct varieties of Ehlers-Danlos syndrome. The disease is most commonly inherited as an autosomal dominant trait. Death from rupture of a major blood vessel may occur in childhood, but most affected persons live at least to middle age.

Homocystinuria

Homocystinuria is a hereditary metabolic disorder involving methionine, a sulfur-containing essential amino acid. The metabolic sequence of methionine normally begins with its stepwise conversion to homocysteine, cystathionine, and cysteine, successively, each step being carried out by a specific organic catalyst, or enzyme. In homocystinuria, the defective enzyme is cystathionine synthetase, which normally converts homocysteine to cystathionine. As a result, abnormally high concentrations of homocysteine and its precursor, methionine, are found in the blood plasma.

Symptoms of homocystinuria include progressive mental deterioration; displacement of the lenses of the eyes; shuffling gait; fine, sparse hair; skeletal deformations; and sometimes fatal episodic obstruction of blood vessels with clots. The joints tend to have restricted mobility rather than hyperextensibility. Death from vascular occlusion secondary to atherosclerosis is common during childhood, but persons with the disorder have survived into their 50s.

Dietary therapy, with methionine restriction and cystine supplementation (cystine is the oxidized form of cysteine) is apparently beneficial in some individuals. Homocystinuria is believed to be transmitted recessively, and thus unaffected carriers of the trait who mate can expect, on the basis of chance, to have one affected offspring out of four births.

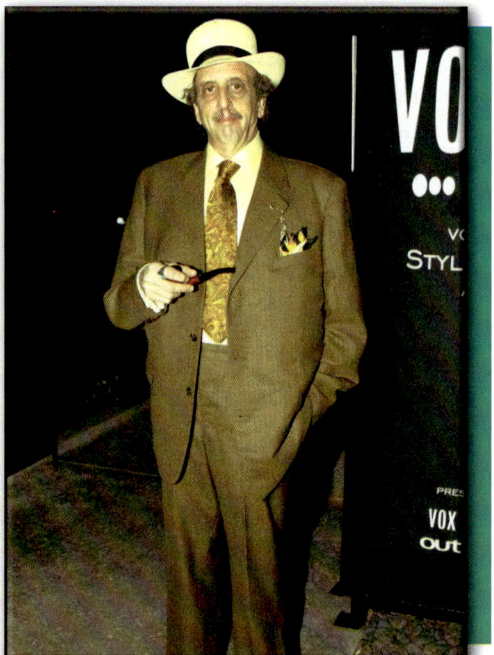

Actor Vincent Schiavelli had Marfan syndrome, an inherited disorder of the connective tissue. Symptoms include elongated limbs, weak joints, and skeletal deformities. Frazer Harrison/Getty Images

Marfan Syndrome

Marfan syndrome, also called arachnodactyly ("spider fingers"), is the most common of the hereditary disorders of connective tissue, having an estimated prevalence of about 15 cases per 1,000,000 population. In Marfan syndrome a genetic mutation causes a defect in the production of fibrillin, a protein found in connective tissue. The main skeletal characteristic is excessive length of the extremities. Weakness of joint capsules, ligaments, tendons, and fasciae is responsible for such manifestations as double-jointedness, recurrent dislocations, spinal deformities, flat feet, hernias, and dislocation of the lens of the eye. Cardiovascular abnormalities, which result from weakness in the middle coat (media) of the great vessels, include insufficiency of the aortic valve and aneurysm (weakening of the wall and consequent bulging) of the ascending segment of the aorta.

Marfan syndrome is inherited as an autosomal dominant trait. No more than 15 percent of cases occur as an isolated instance in a family and may be attributable to a new mutation. Depending on the degree of expression of the trait, affected individuals may die at an early age or may live essentially normal lives. Although the basic abnormality of connective tissue cannot be treated, wound healing occurs normally, and surgical correction of some defects is possible. Marfan syndrome is named for French physician Antonin Marfan, who first described the disorder in 1896.

Mucopolysaccharidoses

The mucopolysaccharidoses include eight or more separate lysosomal storage disorders that, to varying degrees, affect the skeleton, brain, eyes, heart, and liver. The varieties have in common the abnormal production, the storage, and the excessive excretion of one or more mucopolysaccharides (now known as glycosaminoglycans; complex high-molecular-weight carbohydrates that form the chief constituent of the ground substance between the connective tissue cells and fibres). The mucopolysaccharidoses include Hurler syndrome, Scheie syndrome, Hunter syndrome, Sanfilippo syndrome, Morquio syndrome, and Maroteaux-Lamy syndrome.

Hurler syndrome (also called gargoylism, or mucopolysaccharidosis I H) is the most common and most rapidly fatal of the mucopolysaccharidoses. Few children afflicted with it reach the age of 10. It occurs with equal frequency in both sexes, and abnormalities begin to appear when the affected infant is a few months old. Affected individuals exhibit severe intellectual disability, clouding of the corners of the eyes, deafness, hirsutism (hairiness), enlarged liver and spleen, dwarfism with hunched back, short limbs and clawed hands, a large head with wide-set eyes, heavy brow ridges and deep bridge of nose, and poorly formed teeth. The disorder is identifiable within two years of birth, and affected children typically require institutional care and usually do not live beyond adolescence. Death most often results from heart failure, which is attributable to infiltration of heart muscle and coronary vessels with mucopolysaccharides.

Hunter syndrome, or mucopolysaccharidosis II, is a rare sex-linked hereditary disorder that varies widely in its severity but is generally characterized by some degree of dwarfism, intellectual disability, and deafness. The disease affects only males and makes its first appearance during the first three years of life. Many patients die before age 20. Speech and mental development are delayed, the child has frequent respiratory infections, and as the disease progresses a typical constellation of physical signs becomes evident: protuberant abdomen, claw hands, excessive hair growth, coarsening of the face, and retarded growth. The disorder is caused by a deficiency in the enzyme iduronate sulfatase. This deficiency results in a defective chemical breakdown of the mucopolysaccharides, carbohydrates essential in the development of the connective tissues, and a consequent accumulation of mucopolysaccharides in the body, which in turn causes the disease's characteristic mental and physical defects.

Sanfilippo syndrome, or mucopolysaccharidosis III, has three varieties, each caused by a defect in a different enzyme involved in the breakdown of mucopolysaccharides. All three varieties appear in early childhood, and affected persons usually die by age 20. Features of the disease include excessive hair growth and progressive partial paralysis of all four limbs. Mild growth retardation may occur, causing moderate dwarfism, but this is neither as common nor as severe as in related mucopolysaccharidoses.

Morquio syndrome, or mucopolysaccharidosis IV, is a disorder of intracartilaginous bone development that results in severe malformation of the skeleton (particularly the spine and long bones) and dwarfing. The disease is recognized within the first two years of life and is usually progressive until bone growth ceases in late adolescence. The vertebrae of the spine are wedge-shaped and flattened, and back deformity is common. Compression of the spinal cord may occur if back deformity is severe. The heads of the thighbones are small and malformed, sometimes resulting in dislocation of the hip. Knock-knees and asymmetrical development of paired bones are also common. Other symptoms include clouded corneas and circulatory malformations. Individuals with Morquio syndrome have a normal life expectancy. Treatment is directed toward symptoms of the disease.

Maroteaux-Lamy syndrome, or mucopolysaccharidosis VI, is characterized by dwarfism, hearing loss, and progressive skeletal deformity. Onset of the disease is usually in early childhood, with some coarsening of facial features evident by the first birthday. Eye changes, consisting of corneal opacification and hypertelorism, or unusual widening of the space between the eyes, and enlargement of the liver and spleen are also features of the disease. Intelligence is normal, but the lifespan is greatly shortened; affected persons seldom survive beyond age 20. Like other mucopolysaccharidoses, Maroteaux-Lamy syndrome is caused by a defect in one of the enzymes that govern mucopolysaccharide metabolism, which is important in the development of connective tissue. The disorder is inherited as a recessive trait.

Scheie syndrome, or mucopolysaccharidosis I S, is characterized by clawing of the hands, corneal clouding, incompetence of the aortic valve of the heart, and painful nerve compression in the wrist (carpal tunnel syndrome). The disease was described by Harold Scheie of the United States in 1962 and is a mild variant of Hurler syndrome. Persons with Scheie syndrome usually attain normal height and intelligence and can expect a normal life span, which is rare in Hurler disease. Both syndromes are caused by a recessively inherited defect in the enzyme alpha-L-iduronidase, which is important in the development of connective tissues. A related condition is Hurler-Scheie syndrome (mucopolysaccharidosis I H S), which causes dwarfism, progressive blindness, deafness, and heart failure.

Myositis Ossificans

Myositis ossificans is a disorder of unknown cause in which connective tissue and muscle are replaced by bone. In the more common local type (myositis ossificans circumscripta), only one area is affected, and ossification is usually observed to follow injury to the part. In the rare progressive type (myositis ossificans progressiva), group after group of muscles become ossified, until the individual is completely rigid. In this form of the condition, bone develops in tendons, fasciae, and striated (striped or voluntary) muscle. Skeletal growth is normal, although certain abnormalities occur in the majority of cases, particularly shortening of the thumbs or of the big toes or both. Symptoms usually begin in childhood and progress irregularly. Lesions may begin abruptly with local tenderness, swelling, and fever or may develop very gradually, with increasing stiffness and firmness as the only symptoms. Eventually, breathing and swallowing become difficult, and fatal respiratory infections may occur. Steroid treatment of muscle injury and the use of medications to prevent calcification may slow the progression of the disorder. Treatment for the local type may include surgical removal of the bone mass.

Osteogenesis Imperfecta

Osteogenesis imperfecta (OI), also called brittle bone disease, is a rare hereditary disease of connective tissue characterized by brittle bones that fracture easily. The bones are extremely fracture-prone because they are deficient in osteoblasts (bone-forming cells), an effect that appears to be associated with an underlying genetic defect that causes abnormal or reduced production of the protein collagen. There are four types of OI, which differ in symptoms and severity.

An infant with the most common type of OI, type I, is normal at birth, but fractures occur over the following years. The frequency of fractures tends to diminish after puberty. The sclerae of the eyes may appear bluish because of their abnormal thinness, which permits the pigmentation of the choroid (the middle coat of the eyeball) to show. Hearing loss may be caused by deformities of the bones of the inner ear as well as pressure on the auditory nerve because of deformity of its canal in the skull. Double-jointedness, brittle teeth, and abnormally thin skin are also characteristic of type I. In type II OI, the most severe form of the disease, stillbirth is common, or fractures are evident at birth; severe crippling often occurs, and survival to adulthood is uncommon. Type III OI causes symptoms that are similar to type I but is more severe. Type IV OI is moderately severe; it is also similar to type I, but the sclerae are normal.

There is no cure for OI. Treatment is directed toward preventing fractures, controlling symptoms, and developing bone mass. Treatment with bisphosphonate drugs has proved effective in some patients, and the surgical insertion of metal rods in certain bones may prevent or correct deformities.

Pseudoxanthoma Elasticum

Pseudoxanthoma elasticum, also known as Grönblad-Strandberg syndrome, primarily affects the skin, eyes, and blood vessels. The word *pseudoxanthoma* refers to the yellowish papules (pimplelike protuberances) that occur most commonly in the folds of the skin of the neck, armpits, and groin. The colour results from the thickening and fragmentation of elastic fibres in the deep layers of the skin. This causes the skin to lose its elasticity and hang loosely from underlying structures.

Affected persons show signs of poor circulation in the extremities. Leg muscles tire easily, and spontaneous bleeding into the tissues or from any opening is common. Calcium deposition may occur in the skin, and the heart muscles also have many small calcified deposits.

Hence, premature arteriosclerosis is common. Angioid streaks (streaks resembling blood vessels) of the retina are found in at least 80 percent of the cases. Through the ophthalmoscope the angioid streaks can be seen as brown or brownish black bands that resemble the normal retinal vessels but are generally much wider. These streaks are produced by breaks in the elastin-rich internal membrane of the choroid, which permits the choroidal pigment to be seen. Deterioration of vision may occur because of bleeding or degenerative changes. Pseudoxanthoma elasticum is inherited as an autosomal recessive disorder.

Conclusion

The skin and connective tissue of the human body are well-characterized components, whose general structures and functions were described many years ago. Yet, because of the important role that these tissues fulfill in the maintenance of health, they are the subjects of ongoing biomedical research. Of special interest to researchers are the many diseases that affect these tissues, and how these conditions may be detected and treated, or even prevented in the first place.

For the skin, an important area of investigation has concerned the diversity of bacterial organisms that are resident on this tissue and that support its health and enable it to perform its many functions. Millions of bacteria live on the surface of human skin, and understanding how these organisms are affected by genetic and environmental factors is expected to provide much-needed insight into skin diseases ranging from acne and psoriasis to infections and infestations.

The replacement and regeneration of human skin destroyed by burns, wounds, or disease is another area of intense study. Skin stem cells, which give rise to all the various types of mature skin cells, and the ability to revert adult skin cells back to a stem cell-like state, are of particular interest for regenerative medicine. Controlling the differentiation (maturation) of stem cells enables new skin to be tailored to the physiological structure of the skin that originally covered the site of injury. Such sophisticated approaches to skin regeneration are valuable especially in the case of burn victims who have lost much of their original skin cover.

Likewise, connective tissue and connective-tissue diseases are at the centre of several important areas of biomedical research. Achieving a more complete understanding of the complex structure of collagen remains an important goal, and to this end scientists are working to decipher the molecular structure of collagen and how this structure influences its function. Such knowledge could shed light on the growth and development of connective tissue, provide new information about connective tissue disease, and open up new avenues of investigation for diagnosis and treatment.

In addition, the existence of overlap syndromes (e.g., the co-occurrence of two connective tissue diseases in a single patient) and mixed connective tissue disease (MCTD), which is characterized by various combinations of features of lupus, scleroderma, polymyositis, and sometimes rheumatoid arthritis, has raised intriguing questions about the pathophysiology of connective tissue disease. For example, although it is known that MCTD is an autoimmune disorder, why and how the immune system attacks the body to produce the unusual array of symptoms is unclear. Overlap syndromes involving the skin have similarly challenged existing diagnosis and treatment strategies.

Glossary

adipose Of or relating to animal fat.

apocrine gland Any of the large sweat glands that produce both a fluid and an apocrine secretion, are restricted in humans to hairy regions of the body, and are lined by a single layer of tall columnar cells with acidophile cytoplasm.

axillary Of, relating to, or located near the cavity beneath the junction of a forelimb and the body, especially the armpit.

collagen A protein that occurs in the form of fibres, does not dissolve, is found in connective tissue, and forms glue and gelatin on heating for a long time with water.

concatenation Linking together as in a series or chain.

dermatoglyphics Skin patterns, especially patterns of the specialized skin of the inferior surfaces of the hands and feet.

desmosomes A local thickening of the plasma membrane of an epithelial cell that serves to anchor contiguous cells together.

desquamate To peel off in scales.

dorsal Located near, on, or toward the back or posterior part of an organism's body.

eccrine gland Any of the rather small sweat glands in the human skin that produce a fluid secretion without removing cytoplasm from the secretory cells.

glycosaminoglycans Skin materials that absorb and hold great quantities of water.

integument A layer of material, such as skin, that envelopes an organism or one of its parts.

keratin Any of various sulfur-containing fibrous proteins that form the chemical basis of horny epidermal tissues (as hair and nails).

melanocyte An epidermal cell that produces melanin, a pigment that is present in certain animal or plant structures such as skin or hair.

mitosis A process that takes place in the nucleus of a dividing cell and that results in the formation of two new nuclei with the same number of chromosomes as the parent nucleus.

phagocyte A cell (as a white blood cell) that engulfs and consumes foreign material (as microorganisms) and debris.

sebaceous glands Small glands of the dermis, usually surrounding hair follicles, that secrete oils and fat.

subcutaneous Existing or being used under the skin.

turgidity A condition marked by being swollen or distended.

vascular Of or relating to a channel for the conveyance of a body fluid (as blood of an animal or sap of a plant) or to a system of such channels.

ventral Located near or on the belly or lower surface of an animal, opposite the back.

vestigial A small, imperfectly developed body part or organ that is the remains of one more fully developed at an earlier stage or in a past generation or closely related form.

Bibliography

SKIN AND CONNECTIVE TISSUE

An overview of skin biology is found in Ruth K. Freinkel and David T. Woodley (eds.), *The Biology of the Skin* (2001). Arthur Rook et al. (eds.), *Rook's Textbook of Dermatology*, 7th ed., 4 vol. (2004), is a comprehensive work on normal and pathological human skin. Special aspects of the subject are discussed in Howard I. Maibach and Edward K. Boisits (eds.), *Neonatal Skin: Structure and Function*, 2nd ed. (2003); and Joachim W. Fluhr and Peter Elsner (eds.), *Tissue Engineering in Dermatology* (2009). For current research in the field, see *The Journal of Investigative Dermatology* (monthly).

Additional information on connective tissues may be found in James Watkins, *Structure and Function of the Musculoskeletal System*, 2nd ed. (2010). Details on the cellular components of connective tissue are provided in Don W. Fawcett, *A Textbook of Histology*, 12th ed. (1994), chapter 5, pp. 133–169; and Emanuel Rubin and John L. Farber (eds.), *Pathology*, 3rd ed. (1999), chapter 3, pp. 76–103, and chapter 26, pp. 1336–1413.

SKIN DISEASE

Various diseases and disorders of the human skin are discussed in William D. James et al., *Andrews' Diseases of the Skin: Clinical Dermatology*, 10th ed. (2006); Thomas P.

Habif et al., *Skin Disease: Diagnosis and Treatment*, 2nd ed. (2005); and Rodney D. Sinclair, Cedric Banfield, and Rodney P.R. Dawber, *Handbook of Diseases of the Hair and Scalp* (1999).

CONNECTIVE TISSUE DISEASE

A clinically oriented account of connective tissue diseases and rheumatic disorders may be found in John H. Klipple et al. (eds.), *Primer on the Rheumatic Diseases*, 13th ed. (2008). Also of interest are Edward D. Harris et al. (eds.), *Kelley's Textbook of Rheumatology*, 7th ed. (2005); and Emanuel Rubin and John L. Farber (eds.), *Pathology*, 3rd ed. (1999).

Index

D

E

F

G

H

I

J

K

L

M

N

O

P

R

S

T

U

V

W

Y